EVE
Series

Dear Reader,

We would like to start by saying *gracias*—thank you. Simply by picking this phrasebook and learning to communicate with your Spanish-speaking patients, you are showing that you are the kind of caring and dedicated health care professional we want to see in our hospitals and clinics. You share your empathy and understanding of your patients and choose to take the extra step to build a relationship.

We partnered to write this book, each of us bringing our own different stories and motivations. On the one hand, we bring the experience of a Spanish-speaking immigrant who has had to learn how to speak English and navigate the U.S. health care system. On the other hand, we have the knowledge of a health care professional who has experienced firsthand how vulnerable non-English speakers can be when they arrive at the emergency department. We understand the challenges of trying to communicate with patients, who often have to use relatives, even children, to help communicate about serious and confidential issues.

We wrote this book in the hopes that it will help you assess, treat, reassure, and educate your patients, and ultimately help you do your incredibly valuable job—in Spanish!

¡Buena suerte! Good luck!

Saskia Gorospe Rombouts
and Courtney Barbetto

The EVERYTHING® Series

These handy, accessible books give you all you need to tackle a difficult project, gain a new hobby, or even brush up on something you learned back in school but have since forgotten. You can read from cover to cover or just pick out information from our four useful boxes.

 Alerts: Urgent warnings

 Essentials: Quick handy tips

 Facts: Important snippets of information

 Questions: Answers to common questions

When you're done reading, you can finally say you know **EVERYTHING**®!

PUBLISHER Karen Cooper

DIRECTOR OF ACQUISITIONS AND INNOVATION Paula Munier

MANAGING EDITOR, EVERYTHING SERIES Lisa Laing

COPY CHIEF Casey Ebert

ACQUISITIONS EDITOR Lisa Laing

DEVELOPMENT EDITOR Elizabeth Kassab

EDITORIAL ASSISTANT Hillary Thompson

Visit the entire Everything® series at *www.everything.com*

THE
EVERYTHING®
SPANISH
PHRASE
BOOK
FOR HEALTH CARE PROFESSIONALS

A quick reference for medical
and emergency situations

Saskia Gorospe Rombouts
with Courtney Barbetto, RN

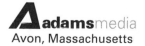

Avon, Massachusetts

An Everything® Series Book.
Everything® and everything.com® are registered
trademarks of F+W Media, Inc.

Published by Adams Media, a division of F+W Media, Inc.
57 Littlefield Street, Avon, MA 02322 U.S.A.
www.adamsmedia.com

ISBN 10: 1-59869-826-5
ISBN 13: 978-1-59869-826-8

Printed in the United States of America.

J I H G F E D C B A

Library of Congress Cataloging-in-Publication Data
is available from the publisher.

This publication is designed to provide accurate and authoritative information with regard to the subject matter covered. It is sold with the understanding that the publisher is not engaged in rendering legal, accounting, or other
professional advice. If legal advice or other expert assistance is required, the
services of a competent professional person should be sought.
—From a *Declaration of Principles* jointly adopted by a Committee of the
American Bar Association and a Committee of Publishers and Associations

Many of the designations used by manufacturers and sellers to distinguish
their products are claimed as trademarks. Where those designations appear
in this book and Adams Media was aware of a trademark claim, the designations have been printed with initial capital letters.

This book is available at quantity discounts for bulk purchases.
For information, please call 1-800-289-0963.

To Darryl and Itxaso, who brighten my world every day.
To my mom for her endless caring and support.

—SGR

To my husband Sal for being my best friend, and my
sons Sam, John, and Andrew, who have brought
me more joy than I could have imagined.

—CB

Acknowledgments

Thanks to Anne Marie, my mom, for her endless caring and support.

Special thanks to Jenny Petrow for her insights and helpful comments, and for being an inspiration to me.

Thanks to the hard-working nurses of Swedish Convenant Hospital in Chicago for their time and support.

Thanks to Lisa Laing for the opportunity to be part of this project.

—SGR

Thanks to Lisa for this opportunity.

—CB

Contents

The Top Ten Spanish Phrases You Should Know

1. **Do you speak English?** *¿Habla usted inglés?*
   AH-blah oos-TEHD een-GLEHS
2. **Do you have any allergies?** *¿Tiene alguna alergia?*
   tee-EH-neh ahl-GOO-nah ah-LEHR-hee-ah
3. **Are you taking any medication?** *¿Está tomando usted alguna medicina?* ehs-TAH toh-MAHN-doh oos-TEHD ahl-GOO-nah meh-dee-SEE-nah
4. **Where does it hurt?** *¿Dónde le duele?*
   DOHN-deh leh doo-EH-leh
5. **How long have you had this symptom?** *¿Cuánto tiempo ha tenido este síntoma?* KWAHN-toh tee-EHM-poh ah teh-NEE-doh EHS-teh SEEN-toh-mah
6. **Please speak more slowly.** *Por favor, hable más despacio.* pohr fah-VOHR AH-bleh mahs dehs-PAH-see-oh
7. **Who should we contact in case of emergency?**
   ¿A quién debemos contactar en caso de emergencia?
   ah kee-EHN deh-BEH-mohs cohn-tac-TAHR
   ehn CAH-soh deh eh-mehr-HEHN-see-ah
8. **Please don't move.** *Por favor, no se mueva.*
   pohr fah-VOHR noh seh moo-EH-vah
9. **Relax. Everything will be fine.** *Relájese. Todo saldrá bien.* reh-LAH-heh-seh. TOH-doh sahl-DRAH bee-EHN
10. **We need the help of an interpreter.** *Necesitamos la ayuda de un intérprete.* neh-seh-see-TAH-mohs la ah-YOO-dah deh oon een-TEHR-preh-teh

Introduction

¡Bienvenidos! If you picked up this phrasebook, chances are that you have come across patients belonging to the fastest growing minority in the United States: Spanish-speakers. Whether you are a doctor, a nurse, or any other health care professional, you have taken an important first step to be able to communicate with your patients.

The next step is to actually use this phrase book and communicate with your patients! Up to now, you may have relied on others to be able to communicate. Family members and support staff are often summoned to translate or interpret for non-English speakers. This compromises confidentiality and increases the risk of receiving distorted information. This phrase book is designed for health care professionals with little or no formal background in Spanish who want to make a difference in these situations. Phrases and vocabulary are organized thematically so they are easily accessible. In most cases, all you have to do is find the phrase you need and read it exactly as it is presented.

In your line of work, efficient communication is key as you deal with health issues and people's lives. In this phrase book you will find phrases and vocabulary clearly listed to communicate in a variety of situations. Have it handy so you can refer to it as needed. Take your time and, if necessary, use the transliterations to make sure you are understood. Questions are designed to elicit simple and clear answers so communication with your patients is not hindered. The goal, of course, is to make sure you get the right symptom and prescribe the appropriate dose.

Keeping all this in mind, don't let it get in the way of your new adventure as a language learner! Communicating in Spanish does not have to be a chore. The key is to have fun. You may initially use this phrase book to look up phrases as you need them. As you continue using it, you will probably find yourself using more and more of the language spontaneously. You may feel warm satisfaction as you say your first Spanish phrase without looking it up. It will be time to take a step further!

Patients will welcome your efforts, and they themselves will be one of the most valuable resources you will have to learn the language. By taking the initiative to communicate in their language, you are showing respect for their culture and experiences as immigrants. Ask them about their countries. Get to know them and their experiences. This phrase book includes sections on how to break and ice and chat with your patients to establish a relationship. These are the types of situations in which you can play with the language and try out new structures and words, which is a key part of the language process. Soon you'll be able to answer with an enthusiastic *¡Sí!* when you're asked *¿Habla español?*

Chapter 1
Communicating in Spanish

In this chapter you will acquire some basic Spanish skills that will help you get started. It is important that you read through it before going to the other chapters, as it will introduce you to pronunciation and basic grammar.

Introduction to Spanish Pronunciation

Are you worried about pronouncing all the new Spanish words? Don't be. Spanish is a phonetic language. This means that—as a rule—each letter corresponds with one sound. The letter *a*, for instance, is always pronounced an open short "ah" sound, similar to the "a" in "cat." This makes it easier to learn. Let's start with the vowels.

PRONUNCIATION GUIDE: VOWELS

Letter, Name	Sound	Example/ Pronunciation
a (ah)	ah	*asma* (asthma) AHS-mah
e (eh)	eh	*enema* (enema) eh-NEH-mah
i (ee)	ee	*cita* (appointment) SEE-tah
o (oh)	oh	*todo* (everything) TOH-doh
u (oo)	oo	*uno* (one) OO-noh

You will see below that there are some exceptions to the rule. The letters *c*, *g*, *r*, and *l* can have more than one sound depending on what letters accompany them. Here is a basic guide to the pronunciation of the consonants.

PRONUNCIATION GUIDE: CONSONANTS

Letter, Name	Sound	Example/ Pronunciation
b (beh)	b	*lóbulo* (lobe) LOH-boo-loh
c (seh)	s before *i*, *e*	*Cecilia* seh-SEE-lee-ah
	c before *a*, *o*, *u*, or consonant	*cáncer* (cancer) CAHN-sehr
ch (AH-cheh)	ch	*parche* (patch) PAHR-cheh
d (deh)	d	*dedo* (finger) DEH-doh
f (EE-feh)	f	*fatiga* (fatique) fah-TEE-gah
g (heh)	hard *h* before *e*, *i*	*gente* (people) HEN-teh
	hard *g* before *a*, *o*, *u*, *ue*, *ui*, or consonant	*gracias* (thanks) GRAH-see-ahs
h (AH-cheh)	silent	*hígado* (liver) EE-gah-doh
j (HOH-tah)	hard *h*	*julio* (July) HOO-lee-oh
k (kah)	k	*kilo* (kilogram) KEE-loh
l (EH-leh)	l	*sala* (ward) SAH-lah

PRONUNCIATION GUIDE: CONSONANTS—*continued*

ll (EH-yeh)	y	*pastilla* (tablet)
		pahs-TEE-yah
m (EH-meh)	m	*mineral* (mineral)
		mee-neh-RAHL
n (EH-neh)	n	*no* (no)
		noh
ñ (EH-nyeh)	ny	*riñón* (kidney)
		ree-NYON
p (peh)	p	*polio* (polio)
		POH-lee-oh
q (coo)	k	*quince* (fifteen)
		KEEN-seh
r (EH-rreh)	hard *r*	*riesgo* (risk)
		rree-EHS-goh
	softer *r*	*píldora* (pill)
		PEEL-doh-rah
rr (dohs EH-rrehs)	rolled *r*	*diarrea* (diarrhea)
		dee-ah-RREH-ah
s (EH-seh)	s	*posible* (possible)
		poh-SEE-bleh
t (teh)	t	*tétanos* (tetanus)
		TEH-tah-nohs
v (OO-veh or veh)	b, v	*vivo* (alive)
		VEE-voh
w (DOH-bleh veh)	w	*whisky* (whisky)
		WEES-kee
x (EH-kees)	ks	*éxito* (success)
		EH-ksee-toh

PRONUNCIATION GUIDE: CONSONANTS—*continued*

y (ee gee- EH-gah)	y	*yeyuno* (jejunum) yeh-YOO-noh
z (seh-tah)	s	*corazón* (heart) coh-rah-SOHN

Transliterations are provided to help you read new Spanish words. How do transliterations work? Just read them as you would read text in English. *Hola*, for instance, is transliterated OH-lah. If you read OH-lah you will notice the silent "h" and the short "o" and "a" sounds. This will give you the support you need to get started. As you interact more and more with Spanish-speakers, you will soon pick up their way of pronouncing words and learn to say them automatically.

Word Stress

Every word in Spanish has one stressed syllable, or accent. Sometimes these syllables are marked by a written accent mark, called *tilde*, as in *clínica*. The pronunciation guide will help you know which syllable should be stressed by marking it with uppercase: CLEE-nee-cah. However, it does not hurt to be familiar with some basic rules about accented words:

• In words that end in a vowel or in the consonants –*n* and –*s*, the stress falls on the second-to-last syllable. For example: *brazo* (BRAH-soh), arm; *cabeza* (cah-BEH-sah), head; *cirujano* (see-roo-HAH-noh), surgeon; *curan* (COO-rahn), they cure; *artritis* (ahr-TREE-tees), arthritis.

- In words that end in a consonant other than *–n* or *–s*, the stress falls on the last syllable. For example: *edad* (eh-DAHD), age; *elevador* (eh-leh-vah-DOHR), elevator.

- Words that do not follow the two previous rules usually carry a *tilde*, an accent mark, on the stressed syllable. For example: *médico* (MEH-dee-coh), doctor; *inglés* (een-GLEHS), English; *dósis* (DOH-sees), dose; *día* (DEE-ah), day.

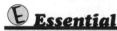

Essential

An accent mark is sometimes used to "break" a diphthong, or combination of two vowels. The word *emergencia*, for instance, has four syllables (eh-mehr-HEHN-seeah), while the word *cafetería* has five (cah-feh-teh-REE-ah). This is, however, is not indicated with the pronunciation guide as it will not hinder communication.

Nouns and Articles

In Spanish, nouns have a gender; they are either masculine or feminine. For words that describe people, the masculine form is used when referring to men, while the feminine form is used when referring to women.

Nouns that Describe People

Nouns ending in –*o* tend to be masculine, while nouns ending in –*a* are usually feminine. Masculine nouns take the definite article *el* (the) and the indefinite article *un* (a), while feminine nouns take *la* (the) and *una* (a).

- *el enfermero* (the male nurse), *un enfermero* (a male nurse)
- *la enfermera* (the female nurse), *una enfermera* (a female nurse)

The general rule to form the plural is to add an –*s* at the end of the noun when it ends in a vowel, and an –*es* when it ends in a consonant. The plural form of *el* is *los*. *La* becomes *las*, *un* becomes *unos*, and *una* becomes *unas*.

- *los enfermeros* (the male nurses), *unos enfermeros* (some male nurses)
- *las enfermeras* (the female nurses), *unas enfermeras* (some female nurses)
- *los doctores* (the male doctors), *unos doctores* (some male doctors)
- *las doctoras* (the female doctors), *unas doctoras* (some female doctors)

There are some exceptions to this general rule, as their ending does not change whether they are masculine or feminine.

- *el/la pediatra* (male/female pediatrician)
- *el/la asistente* (male/female assistant)
- *el/la terapeuta* (male/female therapist)

Nouns That Describe Things

Why is *la cama* (bed) feminine but *el bisturí* (scalpel) masculine? Don't men and women use both? Nouns that describe objects can get complicated, as there is no way to tell whether the word is masculine or feminine. Do not try to reason your way through it. The best way to know the gender of a word is to always learn the word with the article *el* (masculine) or *la* (feminine). This phrasebook includes articles for every new word.

There is a general rule, however, that applies to the gender of nouns. Words that end in –*o* tend to be masculine, while words that end in –*a* tend to be feminine.

MASCULINE NOUNS	FEMININE NOUNS
el estetoscopio . . . **stethoscope**	*la venda* . . . . . **bandage**
el cráneo . . . . **skull**	*la aorta* . . . . . **aorta**
el intestino . . . . **intestine**	*la próstata* . . . **prostate**

But don't live by this rule. There are plenty of exceptions, such as *el diafragma* (diaphragm), and many words end in a consonant: *el paladar* (palate), *la nariz* (nose), *la cavidad* (cavity), *el pulmón* (lung).

Verbs and Conjugations

Verbs in Spanish are trickier than in English. In both languages, verbs are conjugated. This means the verb changes depending on who is doing the action. However, while English has two forms of the verb (see, sees), Spanish tends to have five or more. "I see," for instance, is *yo veo*, "you see" is *tú ves*, and "he sees" is *él ve*. The verb changes according to who does the action that is indicated by the personal pronoun: *yo* (I), *tú* (you, singular, familiar), *usted* (you, formal), *él* (he), *ella* (she), *nosotros* (we, masculine), *nosotras* (we, feminine), *vosotros* (you, plural/masculine; Spain), *vosotras* (you, plural/feminine; Spain), ustedes (you, plural informal and formal in Latin America; formal in Spain), *ellos* (they, masculine), *ellas* (they, feminine).

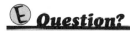

Question?

When do I use *tú* and *usted*?
Both *tú* and *usted* mean "you." *Tú* is used in Spain and Latin America to address friends, acquaintances, relatives (usually younger), or children. *Usted* is used to address someone you want to show a degree of respect to, such as an official, a boss, someone older than you, or someone you don't know well.

Confused? Don't be! In this phrasebook we mainly used the formal forms—*usted* (you singular) and *ustedes* (you plural)—which is what you will use to address your patients.

Here are some verbs you will use in the present tense. The infinitive form ends in either –ar, –er, or –ir. To conjugate it, take the ending out and add the endings below.

REGULAR VERBS

	curar **(to cure)**	*meter* **(to insert)**	*cubrir* **(to cover)**
yo	curo	meto	cubro
tú	curas	metes	cubres
él/ella/usted	cura	mete	cubre
nosotros/as	curamos	metemos	cubrimos
vosotros/as	curáis	metéis	cubrís
ustedes/ellos	curan	meten	cubren

These regular verbs follow a pattern. However, some verbs are irregular and follow no pattern. You will just have to memorize the forms you use the most.

	ser **(to be)**	*estar* **(to be)**	*tener* **(to be)**
yo	soy	estoy	tengo
tú	eres	estás	tienes
él/ella/usted	es	está	tiene
nosotros/as	somos	estamos	tenemos
vosotros/as	sois	estáis	tenéis
ustedes/ellos	son	están	tienen

Alert!

In Spanish there are two ways to say "to be," *ser* and *estar.* The general rule is that *ser* is used with to talk about general, permanent, or physical characteristics, whereas *estar* is used to describe temporary or changeable characteristics. For example, *Soy mexicano* means "I am Mexican" (a permanent state), whereas *Estoy enfermo* means "I am sick" (temporary state).

Every tense—present, past, or future—has its own set of endings. You will see some of them as you read the phrases in this book.

Who Did What?

Unlike in English, in Spanish you don't always have to include the subject in a sentence. In other words, you don't always have to say who does the action: "*I* operate," for instance, can be *yo opero* or simply *opero*. Because the verb is conjugated and has the ending *–o*, we know it is *yo*, I, who operates.

Tips on Communicating in a New Language

Now that you have all the basics, you are almost ready to tackle Spanish. Here are some general tips for communicating with patients in a new language:

- **Memorize short formulaic sentences.** If you remember that *¿Tiene usted . . .?* means "Do you have . . .?" you will be able to ask dozens of questions: Do you have any allergies? Do you have other symptoms? Do you have a problem with that?
- **Use visuals.** Having an anatomy poster you can point to in your office is not cheating.
- **Ask the patient to write it down.** When you don't understand what the patient is trying to tell you, it may help to write it down. However, keep in mind that some patients may not be literate. Don't insist.
- **Use resources in Spanish.** There are brochures and information packages online that you can print and have available for your patients to look at.
- **Don't get frustrated by mistakes.**
- **The goal is communication.** Grammar and pronunciation don't have to be perfect in order to be understood.
- **When the situation is serious, consult a professional interpreter.**
- **Just try!**

Here are some sentences that will help you in tough times:

Speak more slowly, please.
Hable más despacio, por favor.
AH-bleh mahs dehs-PAH-see-oh pohr fah-VOHR

I don't understand.
No entiendo.
noh ehn-TEE-ehn-doh.

Could you repeat it, please?
¿Puede repetirlo, por favor?
poo-EH-deh reh-peh-TEER-loh pohr fah-VOHR

How do you write (spell) it?
¿Cómo se escribe?
COH-moh seh ehs-CREE-beh

Introduction to Spanish Variations

There may be times when you are sure you got the word. You say it. You repeat it. You insist. You get a blank stare. You may have the right word—for one Spanish-speaking region. Just like in English, Spanish has regional variations. You can always ask:

How do you say it in your country?
¿Cómo se dice en su país?
COH-moh seh DEE-seh ehn soo pah-EES

Forming Questions

In Spanish, statements can easily be changed into questions by simply adding questions marks—before and after—and changing the intonation into a question.

You can also form questions using the questions words *dónde* (where), *qué* (what/which), *cuál* (what/which), *cuándo* (where), *cuánto* (how much), *cuántos* (how many), *por qué* (why). Use the word followed by the noun, and—if you choose to add it—the subject.

Where do you live?
¿Dónde vive?

When does Maria come?
¿Cuándo viene María?

What hurts Javier?
¿Qué le duele a Javier?

Most of the questions in this phrasebook are designed to elicit simple *sí* (see) yes or *no* (noh) no answers. If you find yourself in doubt of what patients say, you can ask *¿Sí o no?* (see oh no), yes or no?

Now that you have read about the basic structure of Spanish, you should be ready to start communicating. This phrasebook is organized thematically and by skills. You can read through the chapters and acquire some basic skills in Spanish, or you can go directly to the relevant chapter to access the vocabulary you need most urgently and use it as a reference guide.

Chapter 2
Introductions

An important part of your job is to establish a relationship with your patient. This may be particularly challenging with patients who don't speak English, but it's not impossible. In this chapter you will learn ways to break the ice with Spanish-speaking patients.

Medical Personnel

First things first: Introductions. Patients will probably wonder who you are and what you do as soon as they see you walk in the door. You can introduce yourself using the following phrases:

My name is . . .
Me llamo . . .
meh YAH-moh

I am . . .
Soy . . .
soy

These phrases can be followed by either your first name and/or your title: *doctor* (male doctor), *doctora* (female doctor), *señor* (Mister), *señora* (Misses) followed by your last name. The corresponding abbreviations are *Dr.*, *Dra.*, *Sr.*, and *Sra.*

I am David/Maria.
Soy David/María.
soy dah-VEED/mah-REE-ah

I am Doctor/Dr. Smith.
Soy el doctor/Dr. Smith. (male)
soy ehl doc-TOHR smith
Soy la doctora/Dra. Smith. (female)
soy lah doc-TOH-rah smith

I am Mr. Smith.
Soy el señor/Sr. Smith.
soy ehl seh-NYOHR smith

I am Mrs. Smith.
Soy la señora/Sra. Smith.
soy lah seh-NYOH-rah smith

Alert!

Unlike in English, when you introduce yourself in Spanish you add the article *el* or *la* before titles such as *señor* (Mister), *señora* (Misses), and *doctor/doctora* (Doctor): *Soy la Doctora Sanchez.* (I am Dr. Sanchez.) *Soy el Señor Rodriguez.* (I am Mr. Rodriguez). You do not need to add the article before your first name: *Soy Andrés.* (I am Andrés.)

When meeting a patient for the first time, you can use:

What is your name?
¿Cómo se llama?
COH-moh seh YAH-mah

Nice to meet you.
Mucho gusto.
MOO-choh GOOS-toh.

I'm the gynecologist.
Soy el/la ginecólogo/a.
soy ehl /lah hee-neh-COH-loh-goh/gah

 Essential

Different cultures have different ways of greeting each other. In Spanish-speaking cultures people often greet each other by kissing on the check. However, as a medical professional, stick to a handshake when you meet your patients.

You will find a complete list of specialties in Chapter 3. Here is a list of other medical personnel. Again, there usually are different options for men and women. The general rule is that the word ending in –*o* is for men and the word ending in –*a* is for women.

 Essential

In Spanish, there are two words for doctor, *médico/a* (MEH-dee-coh/cah) and *doctor/doctora* (doc-TOHR/ doc-TOH-rah), which can be used interchangeably. However, only *doctor/a* can be used when followed by the last name, as in *el doctor Pérez*.

MEDICAL PERSONNEL

anesthesiologist . . . . *el/la anestesiólogo/a*
ehl/lah ah-nehs-teh-see-OH-
loh-goh/gah

MEDICAL PERSONNEL—*continued*

cardiologist . . . . *el/la cardiólogo/a*
ehl/lah car-dee-OH-loh-goh/gah

counselor . . . . *el/la consejero/a*
ehl/lah con-seh-HEH-roh/rah

dermatologist . . . . *el/la dermatólogo/a*
ehl/lah dehr-mah-TOH-
loh-goh/gah

endocrinologist . . . . *el/la endicronólogo/a*
ehl/lah ehn-dee-croh-NOH-
loh-goh/gah

gynecologist . . . . *el/la ginecólogo/a*
ehl/lah hee-neh-COH-loh-
goh/gah

medical student . . . . *el/la estudiante de medicina*
ehl/lah ehs-too-dee-AHN-teh
deh me-dee-SEE-nah

midwife. . . . . *el comadrón/la comadrona*
ehl coh-mah-DROHN,
lah coh-mah-DROH-nah

neurologist . . . . *el/la neurólogo/a*
ehl/lah ne-oo-ROH-loh-goh/gah

nurse . . . . *el/la enfermero/a*
ehl/lah ehn-fehr-MEH-roh/rah

nurse's aid . . . . *el/la asistente de enfermero*
ehl/lah ah-sees-TEHN-teh deh
ehn-fehr-MEH-roh

nutritionist . . . . *el/la nutricionista*
ehl/lah noo-tree-see-
oh-NEES-tah

MEDICAL PERSONNEL—*continued*

obstetrician . . . . *el/la obstetra*
ehl/lah obs-TEH-trah

oncologist. . . . . *el/la oncólogo/a*
ehl/lah on-COH-loh-goh

ophthalmologist . . . . *el/la oftalmólogo/a*
ehl/lah of-tahl-MOH-loh-goh/gah

orthopaedist . . . . *el/la ortopedista*
ehl/lah or-toh-peh-DEES-tah

otorhinolaryngologist . . . *el/la otorrinolaringólogo/a*
ehl/lah oh-toh-rree-noh-lah-
reen-GOH-loh-goh/gah

pediatrician . . . . *el/la pediatra*
ehl/lah peh-dee-AH-trah

pharmacist . . . . *el/la farmacéutico/a*
ehl/lah fahr-mah-SEH-OO-
tee-coh/cah

physical therapist . . . . . . *el/la terapeuta físico*
ehl/lah teh-rah-peh-OO-tah
FEE-see-coh

physician's assistant . . . . *el/la asistente de médico*
ehl/lah ah-sees-TEHN-teh deh
MEH-dee-coh

psychiatrist . . . . *el/la psiquiatra*
ehl/lah psee-kee-AH-trah

radiologist . . . . *el/la radiólogo/a*
ehl/lah rah-dee-OH-loh-goh

receptionist . . . . *el/la recepcionista*
ehl/lah reh-sep-see-oh-NEES-tah

MEDICAL PERSONNEL—*continued*

secretary . . . . *el/la secretario/a*
ehl/lah seh-creh-TAH-ree-oh/ah

social worker . . . . *el trabajador/la trabajadora social*
ehl trah-bah-ha-DOHR/lah
trah-bah-ha-DOH-rah so-see-AHL

Alert!

You may have noticed that some nouns for professions, such as *pediatra, terapeuta,* and *psiquiatra,* can be either masculine or feminine. Another exception to the general rule are nouns ending in *–e,* such as *estudiante* and *ayudante.* In both of these cases, the articles are used to indicate gender: *el pediatra* (male pediatrician), *la pediatra* (female pediatrician), *el estudiante* (male student), *la estudiante* (female student).

speech therapist . . . . *el/la terapeuta de lenguaje*
ehl/lah teh-rah-peh-OO-tah deh
lehn-goo-AH-heh

surgeon . . . . *el/la cirujano/a*
ehl/lah see-roo-HA-noh/nah

therapist . . . . *el/la terapeuta*
ehl/lah teh-rah-peh-OO-tah

urologist . . . . *el/la urólogo/a*
ehl/lah oo-ROH-loh-goh/gah

x-ray technician . . . . *el/la técnico/a de radiografía*
ehl/lah TEK-nee-coh deh
rah-dee-oh-grah-FEE-ah

Dealing with Patients

As a medical professional you probably know by now that no two patients are the same. This is also going to be true from your Spanish-speaking patients. It is likely that you will meet people from different countries, backgrounds, and age groups. Everybody will have a different story. Some may speak basic English; others may not speak a word. For some, this may be their first visit to an English-speaking doctor. It is important not to make any assumptions. First, assess the situation. Remember that there are hundreds of possibilities. Here are some useful phrases to get you started:

Do you speak English?
¿Habla inglés?
AH-blah een-GLEHS

I speak a little bit of Spanish.
Yo hablo un poco de español.
yoh AH-bloh oon POH-coh deh ehs-pah-NYOL

I have a Spanish phrase book.
Tengo un libro de frases en español.
TEHN-goh oon LEE-broh deh FRAH-sehs ehn ehs-pah-NYOL

Which do you prefer, English or Spanish?
¿Qué prefiere, inglés o español?
keh preh-fee-EH-reh, een-GLEHS oh ehs-pah-NYOL

Breaking the Ice

Some older patients may come accompanied by younger relatives who speak English. While this may be helpful for communication, remember to address the older relatives as well. You can show them *respeto* (rehs-PEH-toh), respect, by using some basic greetings in Spanish.

Hello.
Hola.
OH-lah

Good morning.
Buenos días.
BWEH-nohs DEE-yahs

Good afternoon.
Buenas tardes.
BWEH-nahs TAHR-dehs

Good evening.
Buenas tardes.
BWEH-nahs TAHR-dehs

Good night.
Buenas noches.
BWEH-nahs NOH-chehs

Most people love to talk about where they come from. Asking Spanish-speaking patients about their country of origin is a great way to break the ice, and it will help you make some of your vocabulary choices.

Where are you from?
¿De dónde es usted? (when addressing one person)
Deh DOHN-deh ehs oos-TEHD

Where are you from?
¿De dónde son ustedes? (when address-
ing more than one person)
Deh DOHN-deh sohn oohs-TEH-dehs

 Essential

In our fast-paced society, at times we confuse efficiency with good manners. However, in many Spanish-speaking cultures, warm and courteous social interactions are highly valued. Spend a few minutes breaking the ice and establishing a relation-ship with your patient.

Remember that in Spanish you have the choice to include or omit the subject. In the first example above, *usted* is the subject, so you could say *¿De dónde es?* or *¿De dónde es usted?* Here are some possible answers:

I am from Argentina.
Soy de Argentina.
soy deh ahr-hen-TEE-nah

We are from Mexico.
Somos de México.
SOH-mohs deh MEH-hee-coh

Another way of saying where you are from is *Soy*, followed by the adjective that describes nationality.

I am Spanish.
Soy española. (female)
soy ehs-pah-NYOH-lah

I am Puerto Rican.
Soy puertorriqueño. (male)
soy poo-ehr-toh-rree-KEH-nyoh

 Fact

According to the U.S. Census Bureau, 64 percent of people of Hispanic origin in the United States are of Mexican descent, 10 percent are of Puerto Rican descent, and about 3 percent are of Cuban, Salvadoran, or Dominican descent.

Note that adjectives describing nationality usually have a feminine form that ends in *–a*, and a masculine form that ends in *–o*. The exception is with adjectives ending in *–e*, such as *estadounidense* (from the United States), which is used for both men and women.

I am from the United States.
Soy estadounidense.
soy ehs-tah-doh-oo-nee-DEHN-seh

In Spanish, adjectives of nationality are not capital-ized. Note also that noun and adjectives need to agree in gender and number. If you are talking about more than one person, add an –*s* for the plural: *peruano* (masculine, singular), *peruanos* (masculine, plural)

We are Peruvian.
Somos peruanos.
SOH-mohs peh-roo-AH-nohs

Dealing with Family Members

There is a strong possibility that Spanish-speaking patients may bring family members as moral support or to help them navigate the system. It is important that you address all of them and establish who is who. Patients may intro-duce their relatives by saying *Este/a es mi . . .* , followed by the noun that describes the relationship.

This is my son.
Este es mi hijo.
EHS-teh ehs mee EEH-hoh

This is Mr. Villa, my father.
Este es el señor Villa, mi padre.
EHS-teh ehs ehl seh-NYOHR VEE-yah, mee PAH-dreh

FAMILY MEMBERS

husband/wife	*el/la esposo/a*
	ehl ehs-POH-soh/lah ehs-POH-sah
boyfriend/girlfriend . . .	*el/la novio/a*
	ehl/lah NOH-vee-oh/ah
fiancé/fiancée	*el/la prometido/a*
	ehl/lah proh-meh-TEE-doh/dah
son/daughter	*el/la hijo/a*
	ehl/lah EE-hoh/hah
father/mother	*el padre/la madre*
	ehl PAH-dreh/lah MAH-dreh
brother/sister	*el/la hermano/a*
	ehl/lah chr MAH-noh/nah
grandfather/	*el/la abuelo/a*
grandmother	ehl/lah ah-boo-EH-loh/lah
grandson/	*el/la nieto/a*
granddaughter	ehl/lah nee-EH-toh/tah
uncle/aunt	*el/la tío/a*
	ehl/lah TEE-oh/ah
male cousin/	*el/la primo/a*
female cousin	ehl/lah PREE-moh/mah
nephew/niece	*el/la sobrino/a*
	ehl/lah soh-BREE-noh/nah
father/mother-in-law . .	*el/la suegro/a*
	ehl/lah see-EH-groh/grah
brother/sister-in-law . .	*el/la cuñado/a*
	ehl/lah coo-NYAH-doh/dah
son/daughter-in law . . .	*el yerno/la nuera*
	ehl YEHR-noh/lah NOOEHR-ah

FAMILY MEMBERS—*continued*

stepfather/ . . . . *el padrastro/la madrastra*
stepmother   ehl pah-DRAHS-troh/
                    lah mah-DRAHS-trah
stepbrother/ . . . . *el/la hermanastro/a*
stepsister   ehl/lah ehr-mah-NAHS-troh/trah
stepson/ . . . . *el/la hijastro/a*
stepsister   ehl/lah ee-HAHS-troh/trah

El padrino (ehl pah-DREE-noh), godfather, and *la madrina* (lah mah-DREE-nah), godmother, are sometimes also considered part of the family. Some people may find support in friends and/or members of their community.

     friend . . . . *el/la amigo/a*
                   ehl/lah ah-MEE-goh/gah
     neighbor. . . . . *el/la vecino/a*
                   ehl/lah veh-SEE-noh/nah
     coworker . . . . *el/la colega*
                   ehl/lah koh-LEH-gah

If patients do not describe their relationship, you can ask:

What is your relationship?
¿Cuál es su relación?
coo-AHL ehs soo reh-lah-see-OHN

Are you relatives/family members?
¿Son ustedes familiares?
sohn oos-TEH-dehs fah-mee-lee-AH-rehs

Extended family plays an important role in some Spanish-speaking cultures. Mexican patients, for instance, may come accompanied by several relatives. You will need to decide what is acceptable for you as far as the participation of family members is concerned. Here are some phrases that will help you communicate your wishes. The verb changes according to whether the subject is singular or plural.

Please wait here.
Por favor, espere aquí. (addressing one person)
pohr fah-VOHR, ehs-PEH-reh ah-KEE
Please wait here.
Por favor, esperen aquí. (addressing more than one person)

Sorry. You cannot be here at the moment.
Lo siento. No puede estar aquí ahora.
(addressing one person)
loh see-EHN-toh. noh poo-EH-deh
ehs-TAHR ah-KEE ah-OH-rah
Lo siento. No pueden estar aquí ahora.
(addressing more than one person)
loh see-EHN-toh. noh poo-EH-dehn
ehs-TAHR ah-KEE ah-OH-rah

We will keep you informed.
Le mantendremos informado/a.
(addressing one person)
leh mahn-tehn-DREH-mohs een-fohr-MAH-doh/ah
Les mantendremos informados/as.
(addressing more than one person)
lehs mahn-tehn-DREH-mohs een-fohr-MAH-dos/as

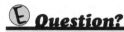 *Question?*

What should I say if people do not leave?
Keep calm and be sensitive to their decision. If they
absolutely must leave, you can explain that it is policy. You can say: *Lo siento. Son las normas del hospital* (loh see-EHN-toh. sohn lahs NOHR-mahs dehl
ohs-pee-TAHL), which translates as "I'm sorry. It is
hospital policy."

You can stay here.
Puede quedarse aquí. (addressing one person)
poo-EH-deh keh-DAHR-seh ah-KEE
Pueden quedarse aquí. (addressing more than one person)
poo-EH-dehn keh-DAHR-seh ah-KEE

Visiting hours are from 2 P.M. to 6 P.M.
Las horas de visita son de dos a seis.
lahs OH-rahs deh vee-SEE-tah sohn
deh dohs ah SEH-eehs

Giving Basic Directions

Whether you work at a large hospital or at a smaller doctor's office, chances are that at some point you are going to have to direct your patients to different places. Pointing always helps, but giving a set of simple directions will mean that you won't send them wandering around. Here are some expressions that will help you point people in the right direction.

What are you looking for?
¿Qué busca?
kee BOOS-cah

Where is . . . ?
¿Dónde está . . . ?
DOHN-deh ehs-TAH

You need to go to . . .
Tiene que ir a . . .
tee-EH-neh keh eer ah

PLACES

bathroom . . . . . *los servicios* (Sp.), *el baño* (Sp., Lat. Am.)
lohs sehr-BEE-see-ohs, ehl BAH-nyoh

cafeteria . . . . . *la cafetería*
lah cah-feh-teh-REE-ah

chapel . . . . *la capilla*
lah cah-PEE-yah

elevator . . . . . . *el elevador* (Lat. Am.), *el ascensor* (Sp.)
ehl eh-leh-vah-DOHR, ehl ahs-sehn-SOHR

PLACES—*continued*

exit	*la salida*
	lah sah-LEE-dah
intensive	*los cuidados intensivos*
care	lohs coo-ee-DAH-dohs een-tehn-SEE-vohs
emergency . . .	*la sala de emergencia*
room	lah SAH-lah deh eh-mehr-HEN-see-ah
main lobby	*la sala principal*
	lah SAH-lah preen-see-PAHL
maternity	*la sala de maternidad*
ward	lah SAH-lah deh mah-tehr-nee-DAHD
parking lot	*el estacionamiento*
	ehl ehs-tah-see-oh-nah-mee-EHN-toh
recovery	*la sala de recuperación*
room	lah SAH-lah deh reh-coo-peh-
	rah-see-OHN
reception	*el área de recepción, la recepción*
area	ehl AH-reh-ah deh reh-sep-see-OHN,
	lah reh-sep-see-OHN
waiting room . .	*la sala de espera*
	lah SAH-lah de ehs-PEH-rah

If you work at a hospital, people may be looking for specific centers. Use *el centro de . . .* to name the center.

cancer	*el centro de cáncer*
center	ehl SEHN-troh deh CAN-sehr
orthopedic . . .	*el centro de ortopedia*
center	ehl SEHN-troh deh ohr-toh-PEH-dee-ah

dialysis center	*el centro de diálisis*
	ehl SEHN-troh deh dee-AH-lee-sees
blood donor center	*el centro de donaciones de sangre*
	ehl SEHN-troh deh don-nah-see-OH-nehs
	deh SAHN-greh

Alert!

There is more than one Spanish option for some place words. Restrooms can be *el baño*, *el cuarto de baño*, or *el servicio* (used mainly in Spain). An elevator is an *ascensor* in Spain but an *elevador* in Latin America. People who have been in the United States for a while may use some English words, such as *el parking* (parking lot) and *el lobby* (main lobby).

Now that you know the names of some places, let's get to the basic directions. The place you refer a patient to may be in a different *piso* (floor).

It is on the first floor.
Está en el primer piso.
ehs-TAH ehn ehl pree-MEHR PEE-soh

It is on the fifth floor.
Está en el quinto piso.
ehs-TAH ehn ehl KEEN-toh PEE-soh

ORDINAL NUMBERS

first . . . . *primer*
pree-MEH-roh

second . . . . *segundo*
seh-GOON-doh

third . . . . *tercer*
tehr-SEHR

fourth . . . . *cuarto*
KWAR-toh

fifth . . . . *quinto*
KEEN-toh

sixth . . . . *sexto*
SEX-toh

seventh . . . . *séptimo*
SEP-tee-moh

eighth . . . . *octavo*
ohc-TAH-voh

ninth . . . . *noveno*
noh-VEH-noh

tenth . . . . *décimo*
DEH-see-moh

Alert!

Some people may get confused by the American definition of "first floor." The first floor in the United States is considered the *planta baja* (ground floor) in other countries, while the second floor in the United States would be *el primer piso*, the "first floor."

After the tenth floor, people often refer to the floor using *el piso* followed by the number: *el piso once* (eleventh floor), *el piso doce* (twelfth floor), *el piso veinte* (twentieth floor), etc.

Now that you know where people want to go, here are some basic directions that may come in handy:

To go to . . . keep straight.
Para ir a . . . siga derecho.
PAH-rah eer ah . . . SEE-gah deh-REH-choh

Go right/left.
Doble a la derecha/izquierda
DOH-bleh ah lah deh-REH-chah/ees-kee-EHR-dah

Go two floors up.
Suba dos pisos.
SOO-bah dohs PEE-sohs

Go up to the twentieth floor.
Suba al piso veinte.
SOO-bah ahl PEE soh veh-EEN-teh

Go down to the third floor.
Baje al tercer piso.
BAH-heh ahl tehr-SEHR PEE-soh

You've learned to introduce yourself, to say what you do, engage in small talk, and send patients where they need to go. The next chapter will address dealing with patients.

Chapter 3
Patients

Can you count to ten in Spanish? Do you remember the word for "name"? In this chapter you will learn to use that basic high school Spanish you may know to manage appointments and help patients fill out medical forms. You will also get the language you need if you have to refer patients to specialists.

Managing Appointments

The first thing the *pacientes* (patients) will need to do is make an appointment. They may call and say *Quiero hacer una cita* (I want to make an appointment). Here are some questions you may want to ask.

Who is your doctor?
¿Quién es su doctor/doctora?
kee-EHN ehs soo doc-TOHR/doc-TOH-rah

Which doctor would you like to see?
¿Qué doctor/doctora quiere ver?
keh doc-TOHR/doc-TOH-rah kee-EH-reh vehr

Are you a new patient?
¿Es usted un paciente nuevo? (addressing men)
¿Es usted una paciente nueva? (addressing women)
ehs oos-TEHD oon/oo-NAH pah-see-
EHN-teh noo-EH-voh/vah

What day would you like to come?
¿Qué día quiere venir?
keh DEE-ah kee-EH-reh veh-NEER

Days of the Week

Here are the days of the week you can use to answer the question *¿Qué día?* (What day?)

DAYS

Monday	*lunes*
	LOO-nehs
Tuesday	*martes*
	MAHR-tehs
Wednesday	*miércoles*
	mee-EHR-coh-lehs
Thursday	*jueves*
	hoo-EH-vehs
Friday	*viernes*
	vee-EHR-nehs
Saturday	*sábado*
	SAH-bah-doh
Sunday	*domingo*
	doh-MEEN-goh

Is Tuesday good for you?
¿Le viene bien el martes?
leh vee-EH-neh bee-EHN ehl MAHR-tehs

What day do you prefer?
¿Qué día prefiere?
hek DEE-ah preh-fee-EH-reh

Months

To ask which date, use *¿Qué fecha?* (keh FEH-chah)

Which date is available?
¿Qué fecha tiene disponible?
keh FEH-chah tee-EH-neh dees-poh-NEE-bleh

To say the date, you will need to know the names of the months:

MONTHS

January . . . .*enero*	
	eh-NEH-roh
February . . . .*febrero*	
	feh-BREH-roh
March. . . . .*marzo*	
	MARH-soh
April . . . .*abril*	
	ah-BREEL
May. . . . .*mayo*	
	MAH-yoh
June . . . .*junio*	
	HOO-nee-oh
July. . . . .*julio*	
	HOO-lee-oh
August . . . .*agosto*	
	ah-GOHS-toh
September. . . . .*septiembre*	
	sehp-tee-EHM-breh
October . . . .*octubre*	
	oc-TOO-breh
November . . . .*noviembre*	
	noh-vee-EHM-breh
December . . . .*diciembre*	
	dee-see-EHM-breh

Numbers 0 to 999

To say the date, you will also need to know the numbers. Here are 0 to 15, which you may need to memorize.

NUMBERS 0 TO 15

0 . . . . *cero*	
	SEH-roh
1 . . . . *uno*	
	OO-noh
2 . . . . *dos*	
	dohs
3 . . . . *tres*	
	trehs
4 . . . . *cuatro*	
	KWAH-troh
5 . . . . *cinco*	
	SEEN-koh
6 . . . . *seis*	
	sehys
7 . . . . *siete*	
	see-EH-teh
8 . . . . *ocho*	
	OH-choh
9 . . . . *nueve*	
	no-EH-veh
10 . . . . *diez*	
	dee-EHS
11 . . . . *once*	
	OHN-seh
12 . . . . *doce*	
	DOH-seh

NUMBERS 0 TO 15—*continued*

13 . . . . *.trece*
            TREH-seh
14 . . . . *.catorce*
            kah-TOHR-seh
15 . . . . *.quince*
            KEEN-seh

From 16 to 19, the number is a combination of *diez* (10) + *y* (and) + the number 6, 7, 8, or 9. For spelling purposes, the *z* in *diez* changes to *c* and *y* changes to *I*, which makes *ci*. For example: *diez y seis = dieciséis.*

After 20, numbers follow this pattern: the tens + *y* + the ones. *Y* again changes to i for spelling purposes. For example, *veinte y tres = veintitrés.*

After 30, the pattern stays the same: tens + *y* + ones, but the *y* does not change and so there are three words instead of two.

NUMBERS 30 TO 31

30 . . . . *.treinta*
            TREHYN-tah
31 . . . . *.treinta y uno*
            TREHYN-tah ee OOH-no

Although you will not need numbers above 31 for expressing the date, knowing them can always come handy to discuss age, money, and other topics. The numbers from 31 to 99 follow the same pattern.

NUMBERS 32 TO 90

32	*treinta y dos*
	TREHYN-tah ee dohs
40	*cuarenta*
	kwah-REHN-tah
50	*cincuenta*
	sin-coo-EHN-tah
60	*sesenta*
	seh-SEHN-tah
70	*setenta*
	seh-TEHN-tah
80	*ochenta*
	oh-CHEHN-tah
90	*noventa*
	noh-VEHN-tah

For 100, use *cien*. For numbers after 100, follow the pattern *ciento* + number.

NUMBERS 100 TO 199

100	*cien*
	see-EHN
101	*ciento uno*
	see-EHN-toh OOn-noh
125	*ciento veinticinco*
	see-EHN-toh veyn-tee-SEEN-koh
199	*ciento noventa y nueve*
	see-EHN-toh noh-VEHN-tah
	ee noo-EH-veh

After 199, say the hundreds, followed by the number.

NUMBERS 200 TO 900

200	.doscientos
	dohs-see-EHN-tohs
272	.doscientos setenta y dos
	dohs-see-EHN-tohs seh-TEHN-tah
	ee DOHS
300	.trescientos
	trehs-see-EHN-tohs
400	.cuatrocientos
	kwah-troh-see-EHN-tohs
500	.quinientos
	kee-nee-EHN-tohs
600	.seiscientos
	seh-ees-see-EHN-tohs
700	.setecientos
	seh-teh-see-EHN-tohs
800	.ochocientos
	oh-choh-see-EHN-tohs
900	.novecientos
	noh-veh-see-EHN-tohs

Dates

Now that you know the names of months and numbers, it is time to say the date. Think backward! Spanish dates usually start with the day, followed by *de* (of) and the month and the year. Note that the article *el* usually precedes the day or date, similar to the English variation "the first of March."

January 2, 2009
el dos de enero del dos mil nueve
August 30th, 2010
el treinta de agosto del dos mil diez

Saturday, December 15, 2011
el sábado, 15 de diciembre del dos mil once

Note that the year is formed by saying *dos mil* (two thousand) and the number. For example, 2009 is *dos mil nueve* (literally: two thousand nine), 2020 is *dos mil cincuenta*, and 2033 is *dos mil treinta y tres*. For years that start with "19," use *mil novecientos* (meel noh-veh-see-EHN-tohs . . .) followed by the number. For example, 1971 is *mil novecientos setenta y uno* (meel noh-veh-see-EHN-tohs seh-TEHN-tah ee OO-noh).

Ⓔ *Alert!*

In Spanish, the days and months are not capitalized. Also, note that cardinal numbers are used in Spanish, although you can use the cardinal number *primero* (first) to refer to the first of the month: *el primero de abril* (April 1). Also, when using numbers to write dates, Spanish-speakers often write the day first, then the month. For example: 7-4-2008 would be April 7, 2008, not July 4.

Time to agree on the date. Use these phrases:

The next available date is . . .
La siguiente fecha disponible es . . .
lah see-ghee-EHN-teh FEH-chah
dees-poh-NEE-bleh ehs

We don't have anything before . . .
No tenemos nada antes del . . .
noh teh-NEH-mohs NAH-dah AHN-tehs dehl

Question?

What do I say if it is a holiday?
If a patient wants to book an appointment on a
holiday, say *Ese día es fiesta. Estamos cerrados.*
(EH-seh DEE-ah ehs fee-EHS-tah. ehs-TAH-mohs
seh-RRAH-dohs), meaning "That day is a holiday.
We are closed." Remember that people from other
cultures may not be familiar with American holidays.

I'm sorry. We do not have an appointment
available that day.
Lo siento. No tenemos citas ese día.
loh see-EHN-toh. noh teh-NEH-mohs
SEE-tahs EH-seh dee-AH

Telling Time

Now that you have set a date, you must agree on the
time. You don't want patients to come late! To ask what
time it is, use:

What time is it?
¿Qué hora es?
keh OH-rah ehs

To tell the time, use *Es . . .* for one o'clock or *Son . . .* for all the other times.

It is 1:00.
Es la una.
ehs lah OO-nah

It is 8:00.
Son las ocho.
sohn lahs OH-choh

Note that the feminine article *la* is used to tell time. Use *y media* for "half past," *y cuarto* for "quarter past," and *menos cuarto* for "quarter to."

It is 1:30.
Es la una y media.
ehs lah OO-nah ee MEH-dee-ah

It is 2:15.
Son las dos y cuarto.
sohn lahs dohs ee KWAR-toh

It is 10:45.
Son las once menos cuarto.
sohn lahs OHN-seh MEH-nohs KWAR-toh

Y (and) is used with the first thirty minutes of the hour, and *menos* (Literally minus) is used with the last thirty minutes of the hour.

It is 9:20.
Son las nueve y veinte.
sohn lahs noo-EH-veh ee veh-EEN-teh

It is 12:40.
Es la una menos veinte.
ehs lah OO-nah MEH-nohs veh-EEN-teh

Now that you know the times, it is time to set up an appointment. To say *At . . .* , add an *A* before the article *el* or *la*.

At what time is the appointment?
¿A qué hora es la cita?
ah keh OH-rah ehs lah SEE-tah

At 4:45.
A las cinco menos cuarto.
OR *A las cinco cuarenta y cinco.*
ah lahs SEEN-coh MEH-nohs KWAR-toh/ah lahs
SEEN-coh coo-ah-REHN-tah ee SEEN-coh

We have an opening at 6:30.
Tenemos una cita a las seis y media.
teh-NEH-mohs OO-nah SEE-tah ah
lahs seys ee MEH-dee-ah

People who have lived in this country for a while may be familiar with the A.M./P.M. system, which in Spanish is pronounced *ah EH-meh* (A.M.) and *peh EH-meh* (P.M.). This system is also used in some countries in Latin America where there is an American influence. However, Spanish speakers tend to use *de la mañana* (in the morning) for A.M., *de la tarde* (in the afternoon) for P.M. in the afternoon or evening, and *de la noche* (at night) for P.M. during the night.

 Alert!

People may have different perceptions of morning, afternoon, evening, and night. In most Spanish-speaking cultures, morning is usually from 7 A.M. until 1 P.M., afternoon is from 1 P.M. until 7 or 8 P.M., and night starts at 9 P.M. Midnight to 7 A.M. may be referred to as *de la noche* (at night) or *de la madrugada* (in the morning/dawn).

Now you are ready to confirm that appointment.

You have an appointment on Tuesday,
March 11 at 10:30 A.M. See you then!
Tiene una cita el martes, once de marzo, a las diez y media de la mañana. ¡Hasta entonces!

Helping with Medical Forms

You are probably familiar with the amount of paperwork that needs to be filled out. Sometimes patients will fill out paperwork themselves, and sometimes you will ask them questions and fill it out for them. In this section, you will learn questions, phrases, and techniques for helping patients fill out their forms correctly.

Basic Information

As you give the *formularios* (fohr-moo-LAH-ree-ohs), or forms, to the patient, you can say:

Please fill out this form.
Por favor, rellene este formulario.
pohr fah-VOHR, reh-YEH-neh EHS-teh
fohr-moo-LAH-ree-oh

Do you need help?
¿Necesita ayuda?
neh-seh-SEE-tah ah-YOO-dah

An effective and easy way to offer support is to tell the patient the Spanish translation of each section. You can use the verb *es* (is). Here are some examples:

"Name" *es* "*nombre.*"
"name" ehs "NOHM-breh"

"Last name" *es* "*apellido.*"
"last name" ehs "ah-peh-YEE-doh"

"Maiden name" *es "nombre de soltera."*
"maiden name" ehs "NOHM-breh deh sohl-TEH-rah"

"Date" *es "fecha"*
"date" ehs "FEH-chah"

 Essential

> People who come from Spanish-speaking coun-
> tries usually have two last names, or *apellidos*, as
> in *David Castro Román*. People get their first last
> name—in this case, *Castro*—from their father, and
> the second last name—*Román*—from their mother.
> Make sure they write their whole last name—no mat-
> ter how long—in the section for last name, as it may
> create confusion otherwise.

Write both last names.
Escriba ambos apellidos.
ehs-CREE-bah AHM-bohs ah-peh-YEE-dohs

Here are other sections patients are likely to find in
medical forms:

SECTIONS

address . . . . *dirección*
dee-rehk-see-OHN
age . . . . *edad*
eh-DAHD

SECTIONS—*continued*

blood type......	*grupo sanguíneo*
	GROO-poh sahn-GHEE-neh-oh
city	*ciudad*
	see-oo-DAHD
date of birth	*fecha de nacimiento*
	FEH-chah deh nah-see-mee-EHN-toh
e-mail, ...	*e-mail* OR *correo electrónico*
email	coh-RREH-oh eh-lehc-TROH-nee-coh
emergency	*contacto de emergencia*
contact	cohn-TAC-toh deh eh-mehr-HEHN-see-ah
marital status ..	*estado civil*
	ehs-TAH-doh see-VEEHL
occupation	*profesión*
	proh-feh-see-OHN
phone	*número de teléfono*
number	NOO-meh-roh deh teh-leh-FOH-noh
place of	*lugar de empleo*
employment	loo-GAHR deh ehm-PLEH-oh
social security ..	*número del seguro social*
number	NOO-meh-roh dehl seh-goo-ree-DAHD
	soh see AHL
state	*estado*
	ehs-TAH-doh
zip code	*código postal*
	COH-dee-goh pohs-TAHL

As you review the form, the patient may have forgotten something. Use these basic commands to help them complete it.

This section is missing.
Falta esta sección.
FAHL-tah EHS-tah sec-see-OHN

Write the date.
Escriba la fecha.
ehs-CREE-bah lah FEH-chah

 Fact

The most common blood types are 0+, *cero posi-tivo,* (SEH-roh poh-see-TEE-voh) and A+, *a positivo* (ah poh-see-TEE-voh). One in every three people has one or the other. One in every twelve people has B+, *be positivo* (beh poh-see-TEE-voh), one in every fifteen has have 0-, *cero negativo* (SEH-roh neh-gah-TEE-voh), and one in every sixteen has A-, *a negativo* (ah neh-gah-TEE-voh). Less common blood types are AB+ (ah bah poh-see-TEE-voh), B- (beh neh-gah-TEE-voh), and AB- (ah beh neh-gah-TEE-voh). The "rh" factor in Spanish is said "EH-rreh AH-cheh."

Quite understandably, some patients may have questions about what they are signing. They may ask *¿Qué es esto?* (What is this?). Use these phrases to explain.

It says you have to pay for our services.
Dice que usted tiene que pagar los servicios.

DEE-seh keh oos-TEHD tee-EH-neh keh
pah-GAHR lohs sehr-VEE-see-ohs

Insurance Information

Next you'll need to know all about the patient's *seguro médico* (seh-GOO-roh MEH-dee-coh), medical insurance. Here are some questions to get started:

Do you have medical insurance?
¿Tiene seguro médico?
tee-EH-neh seh-GOO-roh MEH-dee-coh

How do you plan to pay?
¿Cómo va a pagar?
COH-moh vah ah pah-GAHR

 Essential

As a caring medical professional, you have taken the first steps to be able to communicate with your patients. Be an agent of change! If they don't exist already, insist that your place of work offer forms translated into other languages so people who are not fluent in English can understand them.

Get the details using questions starting with *¿Cuál es . . . ?* (What is . . . ?)

What is your insurance company?
¿Cuál es su companía de seguros?
coo-AHL ehs soo com-pah-NYEE-
ah deh seh-GOO-rohs

What is your policy number?
¿Cuál es su número de póliza?
coo-AHL ehs soo NOO-meh-roh deh POH-lee-sah

What is your group number?
¿Cuál es su número de grupo?
coo-AHL ehs soo NOO-meh-roh deh GROO-poh

Here are some further questions to help make sure you have all the information.

Who is the policy holder?
¿Quién es el titular de la póliza de seguros?
kee-EHN ehs ehl tee-too-LAHR deh lah
POH-lee-sah deh seh-GOO-rohs

Do you have more than one insurance provider?
¿Tiene más de un seguro?
tee-EH-neh mahs deh oon seh-GOO-roh

Do you receive state aid/Medicaid/Medicare?
¿Recibe usted ayuda estatal/Medicaid/Medicare?
reh-SEE-beh oos-TEHD ah-YOO-dah ehs-tah-TAHL

Is it a PPO or an HMO?
¿Es un OPP o un OMS?
eh soon oh peh peh oh oon oh EH-meh EH-seh

 Alert!

Don't get confused by acronyms that you don't rec-
ognize. Sometimes it helps to read them backwards.
PPO in Spanish, for instance, is *OPP (Organización
de Proveedores de Preferentes).* Other times, you
may have to use your imagination: HMO is *OMS
(Organización para el Mantenimiento de la Salud).*

Be aware that some Spanish-speakers may say the
English forms with Spanish pronunciation. HMO would be
"AH-cheh EH-meh oh," while PPO would be "peh-peh-oh."

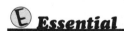 *Essential*

Some people who are new to this country may not
be familiar with how the system works. Be patient.
Try to have as much information as possible available in languages other than English. Some websites, such as CDC's *www.cdc.gov/spanish*, offer
printable forms in Spanish.

Finally, here are some ways to break the not-so-good
news about medical insurance.

I'm sorry. We don't accept this insurance.
Lo siento. No aceptamos este seguro.
loh see-EHN-toh. noh ah-sep-TAH-mohs
EHS-teh seh-GOO-roh

You have a copay of $10 for this visit.
Tiene que pagar diez dólares con su visita.
tee-EH-neh keh pah-GAHR dee-EHS DOH-lah-rehs
cohn soo vee-SEE-tah

Collecting Medical History

From *las alergias* (allergies) to *las operaciones* (surgeries), it is important that you get accurate information about a patient's history. You can start with these basic questions:

Are you taking any medications?
¿Está tomando alguna medicina?
ehs-TAH toh-MAHN-doh ahl-GOO-
nah meh-dee-SEE-nah

Have you ever been hospitalized?
¿Ha sido hospitalizado/a alguna vez?
ah SEE-doh ohs-pee-tah-lee-SAH-
doh/dah ahl-GOO-nah vehs

If yes, for what reasons?
Si la respuesta es sí, ¿por qué motivo?

see lah rehs-poo-EHS-tah ehs see,
pohr keh moh-TEE-voh

Who do you live with?
¿Con quién vive?
cohn kee-EHN VEE-veh

Are you being hurt or threatened at home?
¿Le están maltratando o amenazando en casa?
leh ehs-TAHN mahl-trah-TAHN-doh oh ah-
meh-nah-SAHN-doh ehn CAH-sah

Have you ever had surgery?
¿Ha tenido alguna operación?
ah teh-NEE-doh ahl-GOO-nah oh-peh-rah-see-OHN

Allergies

An important part of a patient's medical history is
allergies. Don't forget to ask:

Do you have any allergies?
¿Tiene alguna alergia?
tee-EH-neh ahl-GOO-nah ah-LEHR-hee-ah

To describe an allergy people may say *Tengo alergia a*
. . . (literally: I have an allergy to . . .) or *Soy alérgico/a a* . . .
(I am allergic to . . .). Use *alérgico* if you are or are talking
to a man, and *alérgica* for women.

Are you allergic to any medications?
¿Es alérgico/a a alguna medicina?
ehs ah-LEHR-hee-coh/cah ah ahl-
GOO-nah meh-dee-SEE-nah

I am allergic to cats.
Tengo alergia a los gatos.
TEHN-goh ah-LEHR-hee-ah ah lohs GAH-tohs
Soy alérgico/a a los gatos.
soy ah-LEHR-hee-coh/cah ah lohs GAH-tohs

Here is a list of other possible allergies:

ALLERGIES

animal allergy	*alergia a los animales* ah-LEHR-hee-ah ah lohs ah-nee-MAH-lehs
antibiotics allergy . .	*alergia a los antibióticos* ah-LEHR-hee-ah ah lohs ahn-tee-bee-OH-tee-cohs
dust allergy	*alergia al polvo* ah-LEHR-hee-ah ahl POHL-voh
insect sting . . . . **allergy**	*alergia a las picaduras de insectos* ah-LEHR-hee-ah ah lahs pee-cah- DOO-rahs deh een-SEC-tohs
peanut allergy	*alergia a los cacahuetes* ah-LEHR-hee-ah ah lohs cah-cah-oo-EH-tehs
pollen allergy	*alergia al polen* ah-LEHR-hee-ah ahl POH-lehn

ALLERGIES—*continued*

shellfish allergy . . . . *alergia al marisco*
                        ah-LEHR-hee-ah ahl mah-REES-coh

soy allergy. . . . .*alergia a la soja*
                        ah-LEHR-hee-ah ah lah SOH-hah

wheat allergy . . . . . . *alergia al trigo*
                        ah-LEHR-hee-ah ah TREE-goh

yeast allergy . . . .*alergia a la levadura*
                        ah-LEHR-hee-ah ah lah
                        leh-vah-DOO-rah

Fact

According to the Asthma and Allergy Foundation of America, 38 percent of all Americans suffer from some sort of allergic condition. Approximately two million people develop severe allergic reactions to insect stings, such as *abejas* (ah-BEH-hahs), bees.

Some patients may be lactose intolerant or aspirin sensitive or may have reactions to different drugs. This is what they may say:

I'm lactose intolerant.
Tengo intolerancia a la lactosa.
TEHN-goh een-toh-leh-RAHN-
see-ah ah lah lac-toh-sah

I get a reaction to anesthesia.
Me da una reacción con la anestesia.

meh dah OO-nah reh-ac-see-OHN
cohn lah ah-nehs-TEH-see-ah

Or they may simply say *No puedo tomar . . .* (I can't
take/eat/drink . . .)

I can't take any aspirin.
No puedo tomar aspirina.
noh poo-EH-doh TOH-mahr as-pee-REE-nah

Family Illnesses and Existing Conditions
It is also important to check for any family history of
conditions and illnesses. Here are some further phrases:

Do you have any chronic conditions, such as high
blood pressure?
*¿Padece de alguna condición crónica,
como la presión alta?*
pah-DEH-seh deh ahl-GOO-nah cohn-dee-see-OHN
CROH-nee-cah, COH-moh lah preh-see-OHN AHL-tah

Do you have a family history of . . . ?
¿En su familia, tienen una historia de . . . ?
ehn soo fah-MEE-lee-ah, tee-EH-nehn
OO-nah ees-TOH-ree-ah deh

SOME CONDITIONS

arthritis. . . . . *artritis*
                ahr-TREE-tees

SOME CONDITIONS—*continued*

asthma . . . . *asma*
AHS-mah

cancer . . . . *cáncer*
CAN-sehr

diabetes . . . . *diabetes*
dee-ah-BEH-tehs

heart disease . . . . *enfermedades del corazón*
ehn-fehr-meh-DAH-dehs
dehl coh-rah-SOHN

high blood pressure . . . *presión alta*
preh-see-OHN AHL-tah

stroke . . . . *derrume cerebral*
deh-RRAH-meh seh-reh-BRAHL

 Alert!

You may have noticed that the names of some conditions, such as diabetes and cancer, have Spanish cognates that are written the same as in English. However, don't expect Spanish speakers to understand when you say them in English, as the pronunciations are very different. If they don't understand you, you can always write them down to convey meaning.

Habits

You will also need to know about some of the patient's habits.

Do you consume alcohol?
¿Toma usted alcohol?
TOH-mah oos-TEHD ahl-coh-OHL

Do you smoke?
¿Fuma usted?
FOO-mah oos-TEHD

Do you take any drugs?
¿Toma usted drogas?
TOH-mah oos-TEHD DROH-gahs

How much do you weigh?
¿Cuánto pesa usted?
KWAHN-toh PEH-sah oos-TEHD

Patients may use the following expressions to answer the questions above:

FREQUENCY

never	*nunca*
	NOON-cah
rarely	*rara vez*
	RAH-rah vehs
moderately	*moderadamente*
	moh-deh-RAH-dah-mehn-teh
sometimes	*a veces*
	ah VEH-sehs
daily	*todos los días*
	TOH-dohs lohs DEE-ahs

Referring Patients to Specialists

There is no Spanish word that fully carries the exact meaning as referral, but don't get discouraged. You can always referred to a referral as to *ese papel* (that paper) or describe it with one of these phrases.

You need to see a specialist in . . .
Necesita ver a un especialista en . . .
neh-seh-SEE-tah vehr oon ehs-peh-
see-ah-LEES-tah ehn . . .

Show this referral when you go there.
Muestre este papel cuando vaya.
moo-EHS-treh EHS-teh pah-
PEHL KWAN-doh VAH-yah

Your appointment is on . . .
Su cita es el . . .
soo SEE-tah ehs ehl . . .

Here is a list of different specialties. Note that you do not need to say the article *el/la* when saying *un/a espe cialista en . . .* (a specialist in . . .), as in *un especialista en nutrición* (a nutrition specialist).

SPECIALTIES

anesthesiology . . . . . *la anestesiología*
                            lah ah-nehs-teh-see-oh-loh-HEE-ah
cardiology . . . . *la cardiología*
                            lah car-dee-oh-loh-HEE-ah

SPECIALTIES—*continued*

dermatology . . . . *la dermatología*
lah dehr-mah-toh-loh-HEE-ah

endocrinology . . . . . . *la endicronología*
lah ehn-dee-croh-noh-loh- HEE-ah

gynecology . . . . *la ginecología*
lah hee-neh-coh-loh-HEE-ah

neurology . . . . *la neurología*
lah ne-oo-roh-loh-HEE-ah

nutrition . . . . *la nutrición*
lah noo-tree-see-OHN

obstetrics . . . . *la obstetricia*
lah obs-teh-TREE-see-ah

oncology . . . . *la oncología*
lah on-coh-loh- HEE-ah

ophthalmology . . . . . *la oftalmología*
lah of-tahl-moh-loh- HEE-ah

orthopedics . . . . *la ortopedia*
lah or-toh-PEH-dee-ah

physical therapy . . . . *la terapia física*
lah teh-RAH-peh-ah

psychiatry . . . . *la psiquiatría*
lah psee-kee-ah-TREE-ah

radiology . . . . *la radiología*
lah rah-dee-oh-loh-HEE-ah

urology . . . . *la urología*
lah oo-roh-loh-HEE-ah

Some patients may not be familiar with these long medical words and may say, for example, *No sé qué es la neurología* (I don't know what neurology is). When possible, explain these specialties using: *Es un/a doctor/a que se especializa en* . . . (It is a doctor that specializes in . . .)

It is a doctor that specializes in the nervous system.
Es un/a doctor/a que se especializa en el sistema nervioso.
ehs oon/OO-nah doc-TOHR/TOH-rah keh seh ehs-peh-see-ah-LEE-sah ehn ehl sees-TEH-mah nehr-vee-OH-soh

You can also explain this as *la ciencia de* (lah see-EHN-see-ah deh), the science of a particular area such as the nervous system.

Neurology is the science of the nervous system.
La neurología es la ciencia del sistema nervioso.
lah ne-oo-roh-loh-HEE-ah ehs lah see-EHN-see-ah dehl sees-TEH-mah nehr-vee-OH-so

You may have noticed the word *del* in the example above. *Del* is the product of joining *de* (of) and *el* (the), so it usually translates as "of the." In cases where *de* is followed by the article *la*, you need to say both words: *de la*.

SYSTEMS OF THE BODY

circulatory system . . . . . . *el sistema circulatorio*
ehl sees-TEH-mah seer-coo-lah-TOH-ree-oh

SYSTEMS OF THE BODY—*continued*

digestive system. . . . . . . *el sistema digestivo*
ehl sees-TEH-mah
dee-hehs-TEE-voh

endocrine system . . . . *el sistema endocrino*
ehl sees-TEH-mah
ehn-doh-KREE-noh

gastrointestinal system. . *el sistema gastrointestinal*
ehl sees-TEH-mah gas-troh-een-
tehs-tee-NAHL

nervous system. . . . . *el sistema nervioso*
ehl sees-TEH-mah
nehr-vee-OH-soh

reproductive system. . . . . *el sistema reproductivo*
ehl sees-TEH-mah
reh-proh-dooc-TEE-voh

respiratory system . . . . . . *el sistema respiratorio*
ehl sees-TEH-mah
rehs-pee-rah-TOH-ree-oh

Now that the appointments and medical forms are taken care of, it is time to learn all about the body parts and pains.

Chapter 4
Body Parts, Pains, and Symptoms

There are more than 100 different body parts where a patient can feel pain. To make the right diagnosis, you'll need to know how to inquire about them. In this chapter you will learn the names of body parts and the terms you will need to assess the situation.

Body Parts

Let's start with the basics: *las partes del cuerpo* (lahs PAHR-tehs dehl KWEHR-poh), the parts of the body. Here are the most commonly used words for body parts, starting with the upper body.

UPPER BODY

abdomen . . . . *el abdomen*	
	ehl AHB-doh-mehn
arm. . . . . *el brazo*	
	ehl BRAH-soh
armpit . . . . *la axila, el sobaco*	
	lah AHK-see-lah, ehl soh-BAH-coh
back . . . . *la espalda*	
	lah ehs-PAHL-dah
breast. . . . . *el pecho, el seno*	
	ehl PEH-tchoh, ehl SEH-noh
chest . . . . *el pecho*	
	ehl PEH-tchoh
elbow . . . . *el codo*	
	ehl KOH-doh
finger . . . . *el dedo*	
	ehl DEH-doh
forearm . . . . *el antebrazo*	
	ehl ahn-teh-BRAH-soh
hand. . . . . *la mano*	
	lah MAH-noh
nail. . . . . *la uña*	
	lah OO-nyah

UPPER BODY—*continued*

skin . . . .*la piel*
                    lah pee-EHL

stomach . . . .*el estómago*
                    ehl ehs-TOH-mah-goh

thumb . . . .*el pulgar*
                    ehl pool-GAHR

wrist . . . .*la muñeca*
                    lah moo-NYEH-kah

Note that the gender of nouns that describe body parts does not change for men and women. *El abdomen* is a masculine noun and carries the article *el*, whether it belongs to a man or a woman.

 Essential

> The word *pecho* is used for both a person's chest and a woman's breast. When referring to breasts, people usually use the plural form *los pechos* (lohs PEH-tchohs). Another commonly used word for breasts is *los senos* (lohs SEH-nohs).

LOWER BODY

ankle . . . .*el tobillo*
                    ehl toh-BEE-yoh

buttocks . . . .*la nalga*
                    lah NAHL-gah

foot . . . .*el pie*
                    ehl pee-EH

LOWER BODY—*continued*

heel . . . . *el talón*
ehl tah-LOHN

hip . . . . *la cadera*
lah cah-DEH-rah

knee . . . . *la rodilla*
lah roh-DEE-yah

leg . . . . *la pierna*
lah pee-YEHR-nah

penis . . . . *el pene*
ehl PEH-neh

shin . . . . *la espinilla*
lah ehs-pee-NEE-yah

sole . . . . *la planta del pie*
lah PLAN-tah dehl pee-EH

testicle . . . . *el testículo*
ehl tehs-TEE-coo-loh

thigh . . . . *el muslo*
ehl MOOS-loh

toe . . . . *el dedo del pie*
ehl DEH-doh dehl pee-EH

vagina . . . . *la vagina*
lah vah-HEE-nah

waist . . . . *la cintura*
lah sin-TOO-rah

Should you use the word buttocks, behind, or butt?
Just like in English, there are several possibilities to name
a certain body part in Spanish. As a medical professional,
your vocabulary choices are clear: always go with the

formal. However, some patients may use colloquial variations that you should be familiar with.

armpit
la axila (armpit, formal), *el sobaco*
(armpit, less formal)
lah ah-KSEE-lah, ehl soh-BAH-coh

stomach
el estómago (stomach), *la tripa*
(belly), *la barriga* (belly)
ehl ehs-TOH-mah-goh, lah TREE-pah,
lah bah-RREE-gah

buttocks
la nalga (formal), *el trasero* (less formal, children),
el culo (colloquial and considered vulgar in
many countries)
lah NAHL-gah, ehl trah-SHE-roh, ehl COO-loh

Basic Commands
Now that you know the names of some of the body
parts, here are some basic commands you can use with
patients.

Move your finger.
Mueva el dedo.
moo-EH-vah ehl DEH-doh

When asking patients to do something, remember that you can always add *por favor* (please) at the beginning or end of the phrase to soften the request.

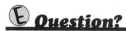

Question?

What should I say if a patient is in excruciating pain?
It never hurts to offer some encouraging words, such as *Muy bien* (mooey bee-EHN), which means "very well," or *Casi hemos terminado* (CAH-see EH-mohs tehr-mee-NAH-doh), meaning "we are almost done." If you need to continue diagnosing, ask *¿Puede seguir?* (poo-EH-deh seh-geer?), which means "Can you continue?"

Lift up your shirt, please.
Levántese la camisa, por favor.
leh-BAHN-teh-seh lah cah-MEE-sah, pohr fah-BOHR

Please, take your shoes off.
Por favor, quítese los zapatos.
pohr fah-BOHR, KEE-teh-seh lohs sah-PAH-tohs

The Head
You have learned the names for upper body and lower body parts. It is time to examine the head. When carrying out an examination, it always helps to warn the patient about what you are about to do.

I am going to examine your head.
Voy a examinar su cabeza.
voh-EE ah eh-ksah-mee-NAHR soo cah-BEH-sah

HEAD

ears	*la oreja* (external)/*el oído* (internal)
	lah oh-REH-ha/ehl oh-EE-doh
eye	*el ojo*
	ehl oh-hoh
lip	*el labio*
	ehl LAH-bee-oh
neck	*el cuello*
	ehl coo-EH-yoh
nose	*la nariz*
	la nah-REEZ
tooth	*el diente*
	ehl dee-EHN-teh
throat	*la garganta*
	lah gahr-GAHN-tah
tongue	*la lengua*
	lah LEHN-goo-ah

More Basic Commands

Here are some additional phrases that will help you examine a patient.

Open your mouth.
Abra la boca.
AH-brah lah BOH-cah

Stick out your tongue.
Saque la lengua.
SAH-keh lah LEHN-goo-ah

Say "aaah."
Diga "aaah."
DEE-gah ah.

Take a deep breath.
Respire hondo.
Rehs-PEE-reh OHN-doh

Cough, please.
Tosa, por favor.
TOH-sah, pohr fah-BOHR

 Question?

What can I say if I'm not 100 percent sure of what the patient is saying?
Did the patient say *pie* (pee-YEH), meaning *foot*, or *piel* (pee-EHL), meaning *skin*? When it comes to getting the right body part, it never hurts to double-check. You can ask the patient to repeat by saying: *¿Puede repetirlo, por favor?* (PWEH-deh reh-peh-TEER-loh, pohr fah-BOHR?).

Common Pains and Symptoms

When a patient comes to you, you may notice his or her expression of pain. To ask what hurts, you can say *¿Qué le duele?* which translates literally as "What hurts you?" The patient may respond with *Me duele . . .* followed by the body part.

Where does it hurt?
¿Qué le duele?
keh leh DWEH-leh?

My ankle hurts.
Me duele el tobillo.
meh DWEH-leh ehl toh-BEE-yoh

My head hurts.
Me duele la cabeza.
meh DWEH-leh lah kah-BEH-sah

For common pains, patients may use a different phrase: *Tengo dolor de . . .* , which translates as "I have a(n) . . . ache."

I have a headache.
Tengo dolor de cabeza.
THEN-goh doh-LOHR deh kah-BEH-sah.

I have a stomachache.
Tengo dolor de estómago.
TEHN-goh doh-LOHR deh ehs-TOH-mah-goh.

I have a sore throat.
Tengo dolor de garganta. (liter-
ally, "I have a throat ache")
TEHN-goh doh-LOHR deh gahr-GAHN-tah

Other common pains are:

backache
dolor de espalda
doh-LOHR deh ehs-PAHL-dah

earache
dolor de oído
doh-LOHR deh oh-EE-doh

toothache
dolor de muelas
doh-LOHR deh MWEH-lahs

When the pain seems too excruciating and the patient
cannot get the words out, you can always use:

Where is the pain? Show me.
¿Dónde tiene el dolor? Muéstreme.
DOHN-deh tee-EH-neh ehl doh-
LOHR, moo-EHS-treh-meh

While some pains may be in obvious places, other
pains may be more difficult to point out. For the pains we

cannot see, patients may describe them in reference to internal organs.

I feel pain around the heart.
Me duele por el corazón.
meh DWEH-leh pohr ehl coh-rah-SOHN

I feel pain around my ribs.
Me duele por las costillas.
meh DWEH-leh pohr lahs cos-TEE-yahs

I feel pain around my lungs.
Me duele por los pulmones
meh DWEH-leh pohr lohs pool-MOH-nehs

I feel pain around here.
Me duele por aquí.
meh DWEH-leh pohr ah-KEE

For Spanish names of internal organs see Appendix A. Sometimes pain is triggered by an action, such as coughing or moving.

My chest hurts when I cough.
Me duele el pecho al toser.
meh DWEH-leh ahl toh-SEHR

It hurts when I swallow.
Me duele al tragar.
meh DWEH-leh ahl trah-GAHR

It hurts when I move it.
Me duele al moverlo.
meh DWEH-leh ahl moh-VEHR-loh

Remember that you can always pose a question by changing the verb in a statement to the second person and adding question marks. In this case, change *me duele* for *le duele*. To find out what actions cause the pain ask *¿Le duele al . . . ?*, followed by the verb that describes the action.

Symptoms

Unfortunately, pain is rarely isolated. Patients often will have multiple symptoms. You can find out whether they have other symptoms by asking:

Do you have other symptoms?
¿Tiene otros síntomas?
tee-EH-neh OH-trohs SIN-toh-mahs

Although there are different ways of posing questions, questions with the verb *tener* will come in handy to find out about different symptoms. You can ask *¿Tiene . . . ?* (Do you have . . . ?), followed by the symptom. Here are some options:

Do you have any blurring of vision?
¿Tiene la vista borrosa?
tee-EH-neh lah VEEHS-tah boh-RROH-sah

Do you have any numbness?
¿Tiene entumecemiento?
tee-EH-neh ehn-too-meh-seh-mee-EHN-toh

Do you have a rash?
¿Tiene un salpullido?
tee-EH-neh oon sahl-poo-YEEH-doh

Do you have migraines?
¿Tiene usted migrañas?
tee-EH-neh oos-TEHD mee-GRAH-nyahs

Do you have frequent fatigue?
¿Tiene cansancio frecuente?
tee-EH-neh cahn-SAHN-see-oh freh-KWEN-teh

Do you have loss of appetite?
¿Tiene pérdida de apetito?
tee-EH-neh PEHR-dee-dah deh ah-peh-TEE-toh

Do you have any swelling?
¿Tiene algo hinchado?
tee-EH-neh AHL-goh een-TCHAH-doh

To ask whether the patient is experiencing difficulty doing something, use *¿Tiene dificultad al . . . ?* followed by the action.

Do you experience difficulty breathing?
¿Tiene dificultad al respirar?
tee-EH-neh dee-fee-cool-TAHD ahl rehs-pee-RAHR

To ask whether the patient feels something in particular, use the verb *sentir* (to feel). Start the questions with *¿Siente usted . . . ?* (Do you feel . . . ?)

Do you feel nauseated?
¿Siente usted nauseas?
see-EHN-teh oos-TEHD NAH-OOH-seh-ahs

Here are other types of symptoms you can check on:

Do you feel dizzy?
¿Está mareado/a?
ehs-TAH mah-reh-AH-doh/dah

Did you vomit?
¿Vomitó usted?
voh-mee-TOH oos-TEHD

Does anything itch?
¿Le pica algo?
leh PEE-cah AHL-goh

Are you coughing a lot?
¿Tose usted mucho?
TOH-seh oos-TEHD MOO-tchoh

Alert!

Sometimes there is more than one Spanish word to refer to the same concept in English. Migraines, for instance, can be *migrañas* (mee-GRAH-nyahs) or *jaquecas* (ha-KEH-cahs).

Describing Different Kinds of Pains

The pain you feel after bumping your head on the door is not the same as a thundering migraine. To ask what type of pain the patient is experiencing, ask the following question:

What type of pain do you have?
¿Qué tipo de dolor tiene?
keh TEE-poh deh doh-LOHR tee-EH-neh

Here are some of the options you can suggest for simple yes or no answers:

PAIN DESCRIPTIONS

Sharp?	*¿Agudo?*
	ah-GOO-doh
Pressure?	*¿Presión?*
	preh-see-OHN
Tightness?	*¿Tirantez?*
	tee-rhan-TEHS

PAIN DESCRIPTIONS—*continued*

Stabbing? . . . . *¿Puznante?*
poos-NAHN-teh

Gripping? . . . . *¿Rasgante?*
rrahs-GAHN-teh

Tearing? . . . . *¿Desgarrante?*
dehs-gah-RRAHN-teh

There is always more to the story. To help the patient describe the pain, ask the following questions:

Is the pain constant?
¿Es constante el dolor?
ehs cons-TAHN-teh ehl doh-LOHR
Does the pain come and go?
¿Va y viene el dolor?
vah ee vee-EH-neh ehl doh-LOHR

How often does the pain come and go?
¿Cada cuánto va y viene el dolor?
CAH-dah coo-AHN-toh tee-EH-neh ehl doh-LOHR

Every minute/hour?
¿Cada minuto/hora?
CAH-dah mee-NOO-toh/OH-rah

Every two minutes/hours?
¿Cada dos minutos/horas?
CAH-dah dohs mee-NOO-tohs/OH-rahs

What causes the pain?
¿Qué causa el dolor?
keh cah-OO-sah ehl doh-LOHR

 Question?

Is there a way to gather information visually?
Have visual references ready. To find out how strong
the pain is, have a scale from one to ten. To find
out how long the pain has lasted, refer to a calen-
dar or a clock. Then all you have to say is: Can you
point to it with your finger? *¿Puede señalarlo con
el dedo?* (PWEH-deh seh-nyah-LAHR-loh con ehl
DEH-doh?).

How long have you had the pain?
¿Cuánto tiempo hace que tiene el dolor?
koo-AHN-toh tee-EHM-poh ah-seh
keh tee-EH-neh ehl doh-LOHR

Have you had this pain before?
¿Ha tenido este dolor antes?
ah teh-NEE-doh ehs-TEH doh-LOHR AHN-tehs

Do you break into a sweat when it hurts?
¿Suda usted cuando le duele?
SOO-dah oss-TEHD KWAN-doh leh doo-EH-leh

What relieves the pain? Show me.
¿Qué alivia el dolor? Muéstreme.
keh ah-LEE-bee-ah ehl doh-
LOHR? moo-EHS-treh-meh

Severity of Pain

To judge the severity of pain, it often helps to use a scale from one to ten.

How strong is the pain?
¿Cómo de fuerte es el dolor?
COH-moh deh foo-EHR-teh ehs ehl doh-LOHR

SEVERITY

Light? . . . . *¿Ligero?*	
	lee-HEH-roh
Moderate? . . . . *¿Moderado?*	
	moh-deh-RAH-doh
Severe? . . . . *¿Severo?* OR *¿Fuerte?*	
	seh-VEH-roh, foo-EHR-teh

On a scale of one to ten, how do you rate the pain?
En una escala de uno a diez, ¿cómo
califica usted el dolor?
ehn OO-nah ehs-CAH-lah deh OO-noh ah dee-EHS,
COH-moh cah-lee-FEE-cah OOS-tehd ehl doh-LOHR

Ten is the worst.
Diez es el peor.
dee-EHS ehs ehl peh-OHR

When do you have the pain?
¿Cuándo tiene el dolor?
KWAN-doh tee-EH-neh ehl doh-LOHR

FREQUENCY

All the time? . . . . . . *¿Todo el tiempo?*
TOH-doh ehl tee-EHM-poh

Occasionally? . . . . . *¿De vez en cuando?*
deh vehs ehn KWAN-doh

Sometimes? . . . . *¿A veces?*
ah VEH-sehs

Rarely? . . . . *¿Rara vez?*
RAH-rah vehs

When sitting? . . . . . *¿Al estar sentado/a?*
ahl ehs-TAHR sehn-TAH-doh/dah

When standing? . . . *¿Al estar de pie?*
ahl ehs-TAHR deh pee-EH

When lying down? *¿Al estar tumbado/a?*
ahl ehs-TAHR toom-BAH-doh/dah

When does it hurt more?
¿Cuándo le duele más?
KWAN-doh leh doo-EH-leh mahs

In the morning?
¿Por la mañana?
pohr lah mah-NYAH-nah

At night?
¿Por la noche?
pohr lah NOH-tcheh

Essential

There are several ways to describe a person's posture in Spanish. People in some Latin American countries tend to use *parado/a* (standing) and *acostado/a* (lying) instead of *de pie* (standing) and *tumbado/a* (lying). However, all Spanish-speakers will understand all options.

Questions and Answers about Symptoms

Just knowing the symptoms may not be enough to make a diagnosis. You need all the juicy details! Here are some initial general questions to ask the patient, followed by specific questions for different symptoms.

Have you taken any medication?
¿Ha tomado alguna medicina?
ah toh-MAH-doh ahl-GOO-nah meh-dee-SEE-nah

What have you eaten in the last twenty-four hours?
¿Qué ha comido en las últimas venticuatro horas?
keh ah coh-MEE-doh ehn lahs OOL-tee-mahs veh-een-tee-KWAH-troh OH-rahs

Have you had this symptom before?
¿Ha tenido este síntoma antes?
ah teh-NEE-doh EHS-teh SIN-toh-mah AHN-tehs

How long have you had this symptom?
¿Cuánto tiempo ha tenido este síntoma?
KWAN-toh tee-EHM-poh ah teh-NEE-doh EHS-teh SIN-toh-mah

Here are possible answers to the question "How long?" *¿Cuánto tiempo?* (KWAN-toh tee-EHM-poh):

One hour/day/week.
Una hora/día/semana.
OO-nah OH-rah/DEE-ah/seh-MAH-nah

Two hours/days/weeks.
Dos horas/días/semanas.
dohs OH-rahs/DEE-ahs/seh-MAH-nahs

A week, more or less.
Más o menos, una semana.
mahs oh MEH-nohs OO-nah seh-MAH-nah

To ask about frequency, use *¿Cada cuánto . . . ?* The patient will most likely answer with *Cada . . .* (every . . .) followed by the frequency of time using *minutos* (minutes), *horas* (hours), or *días* (days).

How often do you get this symptom?
¿Cada cuánto tiene este síntoma?
CAH-dah KWAN-toh tee-EH-neh EHS-teh SIN-toh-mah

Every minute/hour/day.
Cada minuto/hora/día.
CAH-dah mee-NOO-toh/OH-rah/DEE-ah

Every twenty minutes.
Cada cinco minutos.
CAH-dah SIN-coh mee-NOO-tohs

Every hour.
Cada hora.
CAH-dah OH-rah

And now let's get down to the questions you can use to ask about specific symptoms.

Cold and Flu Symptoms

To diagnose whether the patient has *un resfriado* (oon rehs-free-AH-doh), a cold, or *la gripe* (lah GREE-peh), the flu, use these questions:

Do you have a stuffy nose?
¿Tiene la nariz tapada?
tee-EH-neh lah nah-REES tah-PAH-dah

Are you coughing?
¿Tiene tos?
tee-EH-neh tohs

Do you cough up phlegm?
¿Tose con flema?
TOH-seh cohn FLEH-mah

What color is the phlegm?
¿De qué color es la flema?
deh keh coh-LOHR ehs lah FLEH-mah

Do you have blood in your vomit?
¿Tiene sangre en el vómito?
tee-EH-neh SAHN-greh ehn ehl VOH-mee-toh

What color is the vomit?
¿De qué color es el vómito?
deh keh coh-LOHR ehs ehl VOH-mee-toh

Dizziness

It a patient complains of *los mareos* (lohs mah-REH-ohs), dizziness, use the following questions. "To be dizzy" in Spanish is *estar mareado/a* (ehs-TAHR mah-reh-AH-doh/dah).

How long do you feel dizzy?
¿Cúanto tiempo está mareado/a?
KWAN-toh tee-EHM-poh es-TAH
mah-reh-AH-doh/dah

Have you fainted?
¿Se ha desmayado?
seh ah dehs-mah-YAH-do

Do you feel like the room is spinning?
¿Siente que la habitación da vueltas?
see-EHN-teh keh lah ah-bee-tah-
see-OHN dah voo-EHL-tahs

Headaches and Migraines

Use the following phrases to assess *un dolor de cabeza*
(oon doh-LOHR deh cah-BEH-sah), a headache, or *una
migraña* (OO-nah mee-GRAH-nyah), a migraine.

Where is the pain exactly? Show me.
¿Dónde es el dolor exactamente? Muéstreme.
DOHN-deh ehs ehl doh-LOHR eh-ksak-tah-MEHN-teh.
moo-EHS-treh-meh

Is the pain in the same place each time?
¿Le duele en el mismo sitio siempre?
leh doo-EH-leh ehn ehl MEES-moh SEE-tee-oh
see-EHM-preh

Have you had recent head trauma?
¿Ha tenido trauma en la cabeza recientemente?
ah teh-NEE-doh trah-OO-mah ehn lah cah-BEH-sah
re-see-EHN-teh-mehn-teh

What do you do when it hurts?
¿Qué hace cuando le duele?
keh AH-seh KWAN-doh leh doo-EH-leh

Do you experience loss of balance?
¿Tiene pérdida de equilibrio?
tee-EH-neh PEHR-dee-dah deh eh-kee-LEE-bree-oh

What causes the pain?
¿Qué causa el dolor?
keh cah-OO-sah ehl doh-LOHR?

A certain food? Smell? The weather?
¿Una comida? ¿Un olor? ¿El tiempo?
OO-nah coh-MEE-dah, oon oh-LOHR, ehl tee-EHM-poh

 Fact

The National Woman's Health Resource Center estimates that one in every six women between the ages of fifteen and fifty-five experiences migraines, which are often triggered by menstrual and ovulatory cycles.

When dealing with women who suffer from migraines, you can also ask:

Does the migraine occur during or before your period?
¿Ocurre la migraina durante o antes de su periodo?
oh-KOO-rreh lah mee-grah-EEH-nyah doo-RAHN-
teh oh AHN-tehs deh soo peh-ree-OH-doh?

Indigestion

To diagnose *la indigestión* (lah een-dee-hehs-tee-
OHN), you can use these questions:

Do you have a burning pain?
¿Tiene dolor con ardor?
tee-EH-neh doh-LOHR cohn AHRR-dohr

Do you have gas pains?
¿Tiene dolores de gas?
tee-EH-neh doh-LOH-rehs deh gas

Do you burp a lot?
¿Erupta usted mucho?
eh-ROOP-tah OOS-tehd MOO-tchoh

What do you usually eat before?
¿Qué come normalmente antes?
keh COH-meh nohr-mahl-MEHN-teh AHN-tehs

Bowel Movements

Get all the details about *las evacuaciones* (lahs eh-
vah-coo-ah-see-OH-nehs), bowel movements, using these
questions:

How many times have you had a bowel
movement today?
¿Cuántas veces ha evacuado hoy?
KWAN-tahs VEH-sehs ah eh-vah-coo-AH-do

Are your stools hard or soft?
¿Sus evacuaciones son duras o blandas?
soos eh-vah-coo-ah-see-OH-nehs sohn
DOO-rahs oh BLAHN-dahs

Are your stools black or bloody?
¿Sus evacuaciones son negras o con sangre?
soos ch-vah-coo-ah-see-OH-nehs sohn
NEH-grahs oh cohn SAHN-greh

 Essential

There are different ways to describe bowel movements. Formal expressions include *hacer de vientre*
(ah-SEHR deh vee-EHN-treh), *hacer una deposición*
(ah-SEHR OO-nah deh-poh-see-see-OHN), and
defecar (deh-feh-CAHR). A colloquial, yet not vulgar,
expression is *ir al baño* (eer ahl BAH-nyoh), to go to
the bathroom. With children you can use *hacer caca*
(ah-SEHR CAH-cah), which means "to poop."

Is the urine normal? Clear? Cloudy?
¿La orina es normal? ¿Clara? ¿Turbia?
lah oh-REE-nah ehs nohr-MAHL,
CLAH-rah, TOOR-bee-ah

With a strange odor? Bloody?
¿Con olor extraño? ¿Con sangre?
cohn OH-lohr eks-TRAH-nyoh, cohn SAHN-greh

Diarrhea

Here are some questions you can ask when a patient complains of *la diarrea* (lah dee-ah-RREH-ah), diarrhea.

What color is it?
¿De qué color es?
deh keh coh-LOHR ehs

Is it dark brown? Light brown?
¿Es marrón oscuro? ¿Marrón claro?
ehs mah-RROHN ohs-KOO-roh,
mah-RROHN CLAH-roh

Is it green? Yellow? Red?
¿Es verde? ¿Amarillo? ¿Rojo?
ehs VEHR-deh, ah-mah-REE-yoh, ROH-hoh

Is it diarrhea with mucus?
¿Es diarrea con mucosidad?
ehs dee-ah-RREH-ah cohn moo-coh-see-DAHD

Is anyone else in the family sick?
¿Está alguien de la familia enfermo también?
ehs-TAH ahl-guee-EHN deh lah fah-MEE-
lee-ah ehn-FEHR-moh tahm-bee-EHN

Have you traveled abroad recently?
¿Ha viajado al extranjero recientemente?
ah vee-ah-HAH-doh ahl ex-trahn-HEH-
roh reh-see-ehn-teh-MEHN-teh

Constipation

When a patient complains of *el estreñimiento* (ehl
ehs-treh-nyee-mee-EHN-toh), constipation, it is time to ask
these questions:

When is the last time you went to the bathroom?
¿Cuándo fue la última vez que fue al baño?
KWAN-doh foo-EH lah OOL tee-mah
ves keh foo-EH ahl BAH-nyoh

What have you eaten lately?
¿Qué ha comido últimamente?
keh ah coh-MEE-doh OOL-tee-mah-mehn-teh

Does it usually hurt when you have a bowel
movement?
¿Le suele doler al evacuar?
leh soo-EH-leh doh-LEHR ahl eh-vah-COO-ahr

Rash

Do you see *un salpullido* (oon shal-poo-YEE-doh),
a rash, on a patient? Find out more about it using these
questions:

Does it itch?
¿Le pica?
leh PEE-cah

Does your skin burn?
¿Le arde la piel?
leh AHR-deh lah pee-EHL

What type of soap/detergent do you use?
¿Qué tipo de jabón/detergente usa?
keh TEE-poh deh ha-BOHN/deh-
tehr-GEHN-teh OO-sah

After bombarding the patient with all the necessary questions, it's time for some action. In the next chapter, you will learn how to walk the patient through different tests and procedures.

Chapter 5
Tests and Procedures

Imagine seeing an MRI machine for the first time, or experiencing an endoscopy not knowing what is inside of you. Tests and procedures are much more manageable when a caring professional walks you through the process. In this chapter you will learn the language you need to explain the uses of medical equipment and support Spanish-speaking patients through different tests and procedures.

Describing Medical Equipment

If you are about to put something in a patient's mouth, he or she may be wondering what it is. Describing medical equipment can help to put the patient at ease. You can explain procedures in three simple steps: first, what it is; second, what it is for; and finally, what will happen next. Use *Esto es . . .* (This is . . .) to explain what something is, *Sirve para . . .* (It is for . . .) to tell the patient what it is for and *Voy a . . .* (I am going to . . .) to describe what you are going to do next. Here are some examples:

This is a tongue depressor.
Esto es un bajalengua.
EHS-toh ehs oon bah-hah-LEHN-goo-ah

It is for looking inside your mouth.
Sirve para mirar dentro de su boca.
SEER-veh PAH-rah mee-RAHR DEHN-troh deh soo BOH-cah

I am going to put it inside your mouth.
Voy a meterlo en su boca.
vohy ah meh-TEHR-loh ehn soo BOH-cah

This is a stethoscope.
Esto es un estetoscopio.
EHS-toh eh soon ehs-teh-tohs-COH-pee-oh

It is for listening to your heartbeat.
Sirve para oír los latidos de su corazón.
SEER-veh PAH-rah oo-ERR lohs lah-
TEE-dohs deh soo coh-rah-SOHN

I am going to place this part on your back.
Voy a poner esta parte en su espalda.
vohy ah poh-NEHR EHS-tah PAHR-
teh ehn soo ehs-PAHL-dah

Medical Equipment: Doctor's Office

Let's familiarize ourselves with some of the vocabulary that describes the medical equipment in a doctor's office.

MEDICAL EQUIPMENT

adhesive tape/	*la cinta adhesiva/el espadadrapo*
plaster	la SEEN-tah ad-eh-SEE-vah/el ehs-pah-dah-DRAH-poh
bandage	*la venda*
	lah VEHN-dah
bandaid	*la curita, la tirita*
	lah coo-REE-tah, lah tee-REE-tah
blood pressure	*el tensiómetro*
cuff	ehl tehn-see-OH-meh-troh
cold pack	*el emplasto frío*
	ehl ehm-PLAHS-toh FREE-oh
cotton	*el algodón*
	ehl ahl-goh-DOHN

MEDICAL EQUIPMENT—*continued*

crutches	*las muletas*
	lahs moo-LEH-tahs
hypodermic	*la hipodérmica*
needle	lah ee-poh-DEHR-mee-cah
inflatable cuff	*la abrazadera hinchable*
	lah ah-brah-sah-DEH-rah
	een-CHAH-bleh
ice pack	*la bolsa de hielo*
	la BOHL-sah deh ee-EH-loh
monitor	*el monitor*
	ehl moh-nee-TOHR
pipette	*la pipera*
	lah pee-PEH-rah
reflex hammer	*el martillo de reflejos*
	ehl mahr-TEE-yoh deh reh-FLEH-hohs
robe	*la bata*
	lah BAH-tah
scale	*el peso*
	ehl PEH-soh
specimen bottle . . .	*el frasco (de recogida) de muestra*
	ehl FRAHS-coh (deh reh-coh-HEE-dah) deh moo-EHS-trah
stethoscope	*el estetoscopio*
	ehl ehs-teh-tohs-COH-pee-oh
sterilized gauze . . .	*la gasa esterilizada*
	lah GAH-sah ehs-teh-ree-lee-SAH-dah
syringe	*la jeringa, la jeringuilla*
	lah heh-REEN-gah, lah heh-reen-GEE-yah

MEDICAL EQUIPMENT—*continued*

thermometer......*el termómetro*
ehl tehr-MOH-meh-troh

timer ....*el microcronómetro*
ehl mee-croh-croh-NOH-meh-troh

tongue depressor ..*el bajalengua*
ehl bah-hah-LEHN-goo-ah

tourniquet.......*el torniquete*
ehl tohr-nee-KEH-teh

Some patients may not be familiar with some of the measurements used in the United States, such as pounds and ounces. When using *el peso*, the scale, you will probably see the weight in *las libras* (pounds) and *las onzas* (ounces). Patients may ask how much it is in kilos by saying *¿Cuánto es en kilos?* (KWAN-toh ehs ehn KEE-lohs). To convert from pounds to kilos, divide the weight in pounds by 0.45. For example, a person who weighs 145 pounds weighs approximately 65.25 kilos. You would say: *Pesa usted 65.25 kilos* (PEH-sah oos-TEHD seh-SEHN-tah ee SEEN-coh POON-toh veyn-tee-SEEN-coh KEE-lohs).

Uses of Medical Equipment
Here are some verbs you would use to describe the uses of medical equipment. To use them, say *sirve para* . . . followed by the infinitive of the verb. In Spanish, the infinitive of the verb ends in *–ar*, *–er*, or *–ir*.

VERBS

call	*llamar*	
	yah-MAHR	
cover	*cubrir*	
	coo-BREER	
clean	*limpiar*	
	leem-pee-AHR	
examine	*examinar*	
	eh-sah-mee-NAHR	
measure	*medir*	
	meh-DEER	
protect	*proteger*	
	proh-teh-HEHR	
relieve	*aliviar*	
	ah-lee-vee-AHR	
see	*ver*	
	vehr	
wash	*lavar*	
	lah-VAHR	
weigh	*pesar*	
	peh-SAHR	

It is for relieving pain.
Sirve para aliviar el dolor.
seer-VEH PAH-rah ah-lee-vee-AHR ehl doh-LOHR

Explaining Specimen Collections

It is important that patients understand exactly what you
need from them, so they don't have to come back again for

the same procedure. Here are some useful general questions and phrases for common specimen collections.

Can I see the doctor's orders?
¿Puedo ver las instrucciones del doctor?
poo-EH-doh vehr lahs eens-trook-
see-OH-nehs dehl doc-TOHR

Have you eaten since midnight?
¿Ha comido desde la medianoche?
ah coh-MEE-doh DEHS-deh lah meh-dee-ah-NOH-cheh

This test must be done on an empty stomach.
Este análisis tiene que hacerse con el estómago vacío.
EHS-eh ah-NAH-lee-sees tee-EH-neh keh ah-SEHR-
seh cohn ehl ehs-TOH-mah-goh vah-SEE-oh

Did you eat today? When?
¿Comió usted hoy? ¿Cuándo?
coh-mee-OH oos-TEHD ohy. coo-AHN-doh

I am going to send this specimen to the lab.
Voy a mandar esta muestra al laboratorio.
vohy ah mahn-DAHR EHS-tah moo-EHS-
trah ahl lah-boh-rah-TOH-ree-oh

We will know the results in two days/a week.
Sabremos los resultados en dos días/una semana.
sah-BREH-mohs lohs reh-sool-TAH-dohs ehn
dohs DEE-ahs/OO-nah seh-mah-nah

Your doctor will tell you the results.
Su doctor/a le dará los resultados.
soo doc-TOHR/AH leh dah-RAH
lohs reh-sool-TAH-dohs

We will call you with the test results.
Le llamaremos con los resultados del test.
leh yah-mah-REH-mohs cohn lohs
reh-sool-TAH-dohs dehl test

Blood Test

Next, let's look at some common tests. Time to draw
some *sangre* (SAHN-greh), blood, for *un análisis de sangre*
(oon ah-NAH-lee-sees deh SAHN-greh), a blood test. Here
are some useful phases:

I am going to draw some blood.
Voy a sacarle sangre.
vohy ah sah-CAHR-leh SAHN-greh

Roll up your sleeve.
Súbase la manga.
SOO-bah-seh lah MAHN-gah

Make a fist.
Haga un puño.
AH-gah oon POO-nyoh

Don't move your arm.
No mueva el brazo.
noh moo-EH-vah ehl BRAH-soh

You will feel a small prick.
Va a sentir un pequeño pinchazo.
vah ah sehn-TEER oon pe-KEH-nyoh peen-CHAH-soh

Apply pressure here.
Presione aquí.
preh-see-OH-neh ah-KEE

I'm sorry, I have to stick you again.
Lo siento, tengo que inyectarle otra vez.
loh see-EHN-toh, TEHN-goh keh een-
yehk-TAHR-leh OH-trah vehs

Are you dizzy?
¿Está mareado/a?
ehs-TAH mah-reh-AH-doh/dah

You may see needles every day, but remember that
others may not. Some patients may not like *las agujas* (lahs
ah-GOO-hahs), needles. Others may even say "I hate needles": *¡Odio las agujas!* (OH-dee-oh lahs ah-GOO-hahs).
Here are some encouraging words for your patients as you
see them getting paler:

It will not hurt much.
No le va a doler mucho.
noh leh vah ah doh-LEHR MOO-choh

You are doing great.
Va usted muy bien.
vah oos-TEHD moo-EEY bee-EHN

It will be over soon.
Acabará pronto.
ah-cah-bah-RAH PROHN-toh

It's better if you don't look this way.
Es mejor si no mira hacia aquí.
ehs meh-HOHR see noh MEE-rah AH-see-ah ah-KEE

Have this cookie and some juice.
Tome esta galletita y un poco de jugo.
TOH-meh EHS-tah gah-yeh-TEE-tah
ee oon POH-coh de HOO-goh

For some small talk that is guaranteed to distract the patient see the section in Chapter 2 on page 23.

Urine Sample Collection

In Spanish, a specimen or sample is called a *muestra* (moo-EHS-trah). To specify what type of sample you want, add *de* (of): *una muestra de orina* (a urine sample).

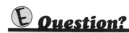
Question?

How do I ask my patients if they want to donate blood?

You can ask *¿Quiere donar sangre?* (kee-EH-reh doh-NAHR SAHN-greh), which means "Do you want to donate blood?" You can also refer them to the American Red Cross site in Spanish for more information: *www.cruzrojaamericana.org*. Say *"Busque la sección 'Dona sangre'"* (BOOS-keh lah sek-see-OHN DOH-nah SAHN-greh) to direct them to the section where they will find information on donating blood.

You need to collect a urine sample in this container.
Tiene que poner una muestra de orina en este frasquito.
tee-EH-neh keh poh-NEHR OO-nah moo-EHS-trah deh oh-REE-nah ehn EHS-teh frahs-KEE-toh

Go to the bathroom.
Vaya al baño.
VAH-yah ahl BAH-nyoh

Clean yourself three times with these wipes before urinating in this container.
Límpiese tres veces con estas toallitas antes de orinar en el frasquito.
LEEM-pee-eh-se trehs VEH-sehs cohn EHS-tahs toh-ah-YEE-tahs AHN-tehs deh oh-ree-NAHR ehn ehl frahs-KEE-toh

Cultures

Although there is a Spanish word for "culture" in this context (*cultivo*), it is not commonly used and patients may not understand if you use it. Therefore, some of the following phrases include a literal translation of the Spanish.

I am going to do a throat culture.
Voy a tomar una muestra de su garganta. (literally, "I am going to take a sample from your throat.")
vohy ah toh-MAHR OO-nah moo-EHS-trah deh soo gahr-GAHN-tah

To do a throat culture, use these phrases:

Open your mouth and stick out your tongue.
Abra la boca y saque la lengua.
AH-brah lah BOH-cah ee SAH-keh lah LEHN-goo-ah

This is a curette.
Esto es una cureta.
EHS-toh ehs OO-nah COO-reh-tah

I am going to swab the back of your throat.
Voy a frotarle la parte trasera de la garganta.
vohy ah froh-TEHR-leh lah PAHR-teh trah-SEH-rah deh lah gahr-GAHN-tah

You may want to gag.
Igual tendrá arcadas.
ee-goo-AHL TEHN-drah ahr-CAH-dahs

It is a normal reflex.
Es un reflejo normal.
eh soon reh-FLEH-hoh nohr-MAHL

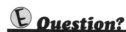 *Question?*

What do I say when we are done?
A simple *Ya hemos terminado* (yah EH-mohs tehr-mee-NAH-doh) will let the patient know that you are finished.

Radiology and Imaging Terms

Here are some radiology and imaging procedures you may have to perform:

COMMON RADIOLOGY PROCEDURES

angiogram. . . . .*el angiograma*
                ehl ahn-gee-oh-GRAH-mah

computed. . . . .*la tomografía computarizada*
tomography (CT)   lah toh-moh-grah-FEE-ah
scan   com-poo-tah-ree-SAH-dah

mammogram. . . . . .*el mamograma*
                ehl mah-moh-GRAH-mah

magnetic . . . .*la imagen por resonancia magnética*
resonance   lah ee-MAH-hen pohr reh-soh-NAHN-
imaging (MRI)   see-ah mahg-NEH-tee-cah

COMMON RADIOLOGY PROCEDURES—*continued*

ultrasound. . . . .*la ecografía, el ultrasound*
                       lah eh-coh-grah-FEE-ah, ehl
                       ool-trah-SOUND
X-ray. . . . .*la radiografía, los rayos-equis*
                       lah rah-dee-oh-grah-FEE-ah, lohs
                       RAH-yohs EH-kees

To protect patients from radiation and possible harm, you may need to ask the patient to wear *un escudo antiradiación*, a radiation shield, which is also called *un protector*, a protector.

Please wear this protector.
Por favor, póngase este protector.
pohr fah-VOHR POHN-gah-seh
EHS-teh proh-tec-TOHR

 Fact

X-rays are safe. To learn facts about safety in radiology procedures, you can refer your Spanish-speaking patients to the Spanish website *www.radiologyinfo.org/sp*.

X-Rays
The phrases in this section are specific to each test. They will help you make sure the test is done in

an efficient and safe way. To specify the type of X-ray you need to take, use *una radiografía* followed by the preposition *de* (of) and the possessive *su* (your). *Una radiografía de su brazo*, for instance, would be an X-ray of your arm.

We need to do an X-ray of your foot.
Tenemos que hacer una radiografía de su pie.
teh-NEH-mohs keh ah-SEHR OO-nah rah-dee-oh-grah-FEE-ah deh soo pee-EH

You need to stand here.
Tiene que quedarse aquí.
tee-EH-neh keh keh-DAHR-seh ah-KEE

Don't move.
No se mueva.
noh seh moo-EH-vah

MRI and CT Scan

Although the Spanish for MRI is *la imagen por resonancia magnética*, some patients may know it as simply *MRI* (EH-meh EH-rreh ee), as a translation of the English acronym. CT scans may be known as *la tomografía computarizada* or *la exploración TAC* (eks-ploh-rah-see-OHN teh ah seh). Both tests require similar preparation. Some patients may not be familiar with either, so you may have to explain what they are.

An MRI is used to see inside the body in detail.
El MRI se usa para ver dentro del cuerpo con detalle.
ehl EH-meh EH-rreh ee seh OO-sah PAH-rah vehr
DEHN-troh dehl coo-EHR-poh cohn deh-TAH-yeh

Please remove all jewelry.
Por favor, quítese todas las joyas.
pohr fah-VOHR, KEE-teh-seh TOH-dahs
lahs HOH-yahs

Lay down here.
Túmbese aquí.
TOOM-beh-seh ah-KEE

We are going to inject you with some contrast
material.
Le vamos a inyectar un material de contraste.
leh VAH-mohs ah een-yehk-TAHR oon mah-
teh-ree-AHL deh cohn-TRAHS-teh

The contrast material may make you feel flushed
for about five minutes.
*El material de contraste hará sentir un
calentamiento durante cinco minutos.*
ehl mah-teh-ree-AHL deh cohn-TRAHS-teh leh
ah-RAH sehn-TEER oon cah-lehn-tah-mee-EHN-toh
doo-RAHN-teh SEEN-coh mee-NOO-tohs

You will go in and stay inside for five minutes.
Entrará y se quedará dentro cinco minutos.

ehn-trah-RAH ee seh keh-dah-RAH DEHN-troh
SEEN-coh mee-NOO-tohs

It is important that you do not move.
Es importante que no se mueva.
ehs eem-pohr-TAHN-teh keh noh seh moo-EH-vah

We are going to strap you.
Le vamos a atar.
leh VAH-mohs ah ah-TAHR

You will not feel any pain.
No sentirá dolor.
noh sehn-tee-RAH doh-LOHR

Keep in mind that MRIs and CT scans can be quite intimidating. To help alleviate a patient's possible fears, use these phrases:

Relax and breath more slowly.
Relájese y respire más despacio.
reh-LAH-heh-seh ee rehs-PEE-reh mahs
dehs-PAH-see-oh

Try to think of a place you love.
Intente pensar en un lugar que le encante.
een-TEHN-teh pehn-SAHR eh noon looh-GAHR keh
leh ehn-CAHNT-teh

Are you claustrophobic?
¿Tiene usted claustrofobia?
tee-EH-neh oos-TEHD clah-oos-troh-FOH-bee-ah

Would you like a mild sedative?
¿Quiere un sedante suave?
kee-EH-reh oon seh-DAHN-teh soo-AH-veh

Would you like some earplugs?
¿Quiere unos tapones para los oídos?
kee-EH-reh OO-nohs tah-POH-nehs
PAH-rah lohs oh-EE-dohs

Alert!

It is possible that some patients who have lived in
the United States for some time may mix Spanish
and English while speaking. This may happen especially when referring to terms such as MRI, which
they may have learned in English.

I can communicate with you at all times.
Nos podemos comunicar todo el rato.
nohs poh-DEH-mohs coh-moo-nee-CAHR
TOH-doh ehl RAH-toh

Ultrasound

An ultrasound is called *un test de ultrasonido, una
ecografía*, or *un ultrasound*. You can do an ultrasound of

el seno (breast), *la tripa* (stomach area), and *la tripa de la mujer embarazada* (a pregnant woman's abdomen).

I am going to put some gel on you.
Voy a poner un poco de gel sobre usted.
vohy ah poh-NEHR oon POH-coh
de hehl SOH-breh oos-TEHD

I am going to put this on your abdomen.
Voy a poner esto sobre su tripa.
vohy ah poh-NEHR EHS-toh SOH-breh soo TREE-pah

 Question?

Should I tell the patient the sex of the baby?
If you don't know whether the patient wants to know this, ask before telling her! Ask *¿Quiero saber si es niño o niña?* (kee-EH-reh sah-BEHR see ehs NEE-nyoh o NEE-nay?)—do you want to know if it's a boy or a girl?

Mammogram

Use the following phrases to do *una mamografía* (OO-nah mah-moh-grah-FEE-ah), a mammogram.

Please put your breast here.
Por favor, ponga su seno aquí.
pohr fah-VOHR, POHN-gah soo SEH-noh ah-KEE

It's going to feel tight.
Va a sentir presión.
vah ah sehn-TEER preh-see-OHN

It will only last a minute.
Sólo durará un minuto.
SOH-loh doo-rah-RAH oon mee-NOO-toh

Don't move, and stop breathing.
No se mueva, y deje de respirar.
noh seh moo-EH-vah ee DEH-heh deh rehs-pee-RAHR

Fact

To learn all the facts about màmmograms, you can
refer your Spanish-speaking patients to the National
Cancer Institute's website in Spanish *www.cancer
.gov/espanol.* Say: *Vaya a la página www.cancer.gov/
espanol.* (VAH-yah ah lah PAH-hee-nah DOH-bleh
OO-veh DOH-bleh OO-veh DOH-bleh OO-veh CAN-
sehr POON-toh gohv BAH-rrah ehs-pah-NYOHL.)

You can breathe now.
Ya puede respirar.
yah poo-EH-deh rehs-pee-RAHR

Are you nursing?
¿Está dando de mamar?
ehs-TAH DAHN-doh deh mah-MAHR

Empty your breast with this pump.
Vacíe su seno con esta bomba de pecho.
vah-SEE-eh soo SEH-noh cohn EHS-
tah BOHM-bah deh PEH-choh

Sharing the Results

Time to share *los resultados* (lohs reh-sool-TAH-dohs),
the results. They may be *positivos* (poh-see-TEE-vohs),
positive, or *negativos* (neh-gah-TEE-vohs), negative. Note
that both words end in –*os* to match the masculine plural
noun *resultados*.

The results are negative.
Los resultados son negativos.
lohs reh-sool-TAH-dohs soh neh-gah-TEE-vohs

There is a problem here.
Hay un problema aquí.
ah-EE oon proh-BLEH-mah AH-kee

Procedures Performed in a Physician's Office

There are several tests and procedures that are usually
performed at a physician's office. From the routine blood
pressure measurement to a basic neurological exam, it is
always a good idea to let the patient know what you are
doing. You will also need to let the patient know what he
or she needs to do to prepare for the test. Here are some
general commands to make sure the patient is ready and
dressed appropriately:

Take your clothes off and put on this robe.
Quítese la ropa y póngase esta bata.
KEE-teh-seh lah ROH-pah ee POHN-
gah-seh EHS-tah BAH-tah

Take your clothes off from the waist up.
Quítese la ropa de la cintura para arriba.
KEE-teh-seh lah ROH-pah deh lah seen-
TOO-rah PAH-rah ah-REE-bah

Take your clothes off from the waist down.
Quítese la ropa de la cintura para abajo.
KEE-teh-seh lah ROH-pah deh lah seen-
TOO-rah PAH-rah ah-BAH-hoh

Remember that you can always sound gentler by adding *por favor* (please) to the request.

Taking a Blood Pressure Measurement

In Spanish, blood pressure is *la tensión sanguínea*
(lah tehn-see-OHN sahn-GHEE-neh-ah), *la presión arterial*
(lah preh-see-OHN ahr-teh-ree-AHL), or simply *la tensión*
or *la presión*.

I am going to take your blood pressure.
Voy a tomarle la tensión.
voht ah toh-MAHR-leh lah tehn-see-OHN

Roll up your sleeve, please.
Por favor, súbase la manga.
pohr fah-VOHR SOO-bah-seh lah MAHN-gah

Your blood pressure is normal.
Tiene la tensión normal.
tee-EH-neh lah tehn-see-OHN NOHR-mahl

Your blood pressure is high/low.
Tiene la tensión alta/baja.
tee-EHN-neh lah tehn-see-OHN BAH-hah

Your pressure is 120 over 60.
Su tensión es 120, 60.
soo tehn-see-OHN ehs see-EHN-toh
veh-EEN-teh, seh-SEHN-tah

Be aware that in some countries, such as Spain, numbers 1 to 10 are used to describe blood pressure, as opposed to 10 to 200.

Taking a Temperature Reading

In Spanish, to take someone's temperature is *tomarle la temperatura a alguien*, and to have a temperature/fever is *tener fiebre*.

I am going to take your temperature.
Voy a tomarle la temperatura.
vohy a toh-MAHR-leh lah tehm-peh-rah-TOO-rah

I am going to put the thermometer in your mouth.
Voy a ponerle el termómetro en la boca.
vohy a poh-NEHR-leh ehl tehr-MOH-
meh-troh ehn lah BOH-cah

Keep the thermometer under your tongue.
Mantenga el termómetro debajo de la lengua.
mahn-TEHN-gah ehl tehr-MOH-meh-troh
deh-BAH-hoh deh lah LEHN-goo-ah

You don't have a fever.
No tiene usted fiebre.
noh tee-EH-neh oos-TEHD fee-EH-breh

Alert!

Patients from other countries may not be familiar with thermometers in degrees Fahrenheit. Have a conversion chart handy as reference. The normal body temperature of a healthy resting adult is around 98.6 degrees Fahrenheit, which is 37 degrees Celsius.

You have a temperature of . . .
Tiene usted . . . de fiebre.
tee-EH-neh oss-TEHD . . . deh fee-EH-breh

Basic Neurological Test

If a patient seems disoriented, you may want to do a quick neurological exam by asking some basic questions.

What is your name?
¿Cómo se llama?
COH-moh seh YAH-mah

Where are we?
¿Dónde estamos?
DOHN-deh ehs-TAH-mohs

What's today's date?
¿Qué fecha es hoy?
keh FEH-chah ehs oh-ee

Follow this with your eyes as I move it.
Siga esto con sus ojos mientras yo lo muevo.
SEE-gah EHS-toh cohn soos OH-hohs mee-
EHN-trahs yoh loh moo-EH-voh

Skin Test

When you are doing a skin test or *un examen de piel* (oon eh-KSAH-mehn de pee-EHL) to diagnose *tuberculosis* (too-behr-coo-LOH-sees), tuberculosis; *alergias* (ah-LEHR-hee-ahs), allergies; or *cáncer de piel* (CAHN-sehr deh pee-EHL), skin cancer, you can use the following phrases:

I am going to examine the skin on your body.
Voy a examinarle la piel del cuerpo.
vohy ah eh-ksah-mee-NAHR-leh lah
pee-EHL dehl KWER-poh

Here are some more verbs you may find useful:

ACTIONS

examine	*.examinar*	
	eh-ksah-mee-NAHR	
measure	*. medir*	
	meh-DEER	
pressure	*.presionar*	
	preh-see-OH-nahr	
touch	*.tocar*	
	toh-CAHR	
weigh	*.pesar*	
	peh-SAHR	

Hospital Procedures

Are you ready for some long words? Here are some of the procedures that will take place at a hospital. You can announce them with *Tenemos que hacer un/a . . .* (We have to do a . . .) Remember to use *un* for masculine words that take *el* and *una* with feminine words that take *la.*

PROCEDURES

bronchoscopy	*.la broncoscopia*	
	lah brohn-cohs-COH-pee-ah	
EEG	*.el electroencefalograma*	
	ehl eh-lec-troh-ehn-seh-fah-loh-GRAH-mah	
EKG or ECG	*.el electrocardiograma*	
	ehl eh-lec-troh-cahr-dee-oh-GRAH-mah	

PROCEDURES—*continued*

endoscopy . . . . *la endoscopia*
             lah ehn-dohs-COH-pee-ah

When you share some of these long words with patients you may get a blank stare. You will probably have to explain what these tests are and how they are performed. Here are some useful phrases. You will first find some general phrases that can be used for all of the tests, followed by specific phrases for each test.

It is a minimally invasive test/procedure.
Es un test/procedimiento mínimamente invasivo.
eh soon test/proh-seh-dee-mee-EHN-toh MEE-nee-mah-mehn-teh een-vah-SEE-voh

The test lasts ten minutes.
El test dura veinte minutos.
ehls test doo-rah-RAH VEYN-teh mee-NOO-tohs

The risks are minimal.
El riesgo es mínimo.
ehl ree-EHS-goh ehs MEE-nee-moh

POSSIBLE RISKS

allergic reactions . . *las reacciones alérgicas*
               lahs reh-ahc-see-OH-nehs
               ah-LEHR-hee-cahs
infection . . . . *la infección*
               lah een-fehc-see-OHN

POSSIBLE RISKS—*continued*

over-sedation . . . . .*la sedación excesiva*
                 lah seh-dah-see-OHN eks-seh-SEE-vah

punctured organs. .*las perforaciones en los órganos*
                 lahs pehr-foh-rah-see-OH-nehs ehn
                 lohs OHR-gah-nohs

EKG, ECG, or Electrocardiogram

If you are concerned about *enfermedades cardiovas-culares* (ehn-fehr-meh-DAH-dehs cahr-dee-oh-vahs-coo-LAH-rehs), cardiovascular illnesses, you may have to do *un electrocardiograma* (oon eh-lec-troh-cahr-dee-oh-GRAH-mah), an electrocardiogram.

It is a test that measures the electrical activity
of the heart.
Es un test que mide la actividad eléctrica del corazón.
ehs oon test keh MEE-deh lah ahc-tee-vee-DAHD
eh-LEC-tree-cah dehl coh-rah-SOHN

I am going to put these electrodes on your
chest, arms, and legs.
*Voy a ponerle estos electrodos en el pecho,
los brazos y las piernas.*
vohy ah poh-NEHR-leh EHS-tohs eh-lec-TROH-dohs
ehn ehl PEH-choh, lohs BRAH-sohs ee lahs
pee-EHR-nahs

EEG

When you need to look at *la actividad del cerebro*, brain activity, it is time for *un electroencefalograma* (oon eh-lec-troh-ehn-seh-fah-loh-GRAH-mah), an EEG. This test is often used to see if a patient has *ataques* (ah-TAH-kehs), seizures.

It is a test that measures the electrical activity produced by the brain.
Es un test que mide la actividad eléctrica producida por el cerebro.
ehs oon test keh MEE-dah lah ahc-tee-vee-DAHD proh-doo-SEE-dah pohr ehl seh-REH-broh

I am going to put some electrodes on your head.
Voy a poner unos electrodos en su cabeza.
vohy ah poh-NEHR OO-nohs eh-lec-TROH-dohs ehn soo cah-BEH-sah

The monitor will measure the activity.
El monitor medirá la actividad.
chls moh nee TOHR meh-dee-RAH lah ahc-tee-vee-DAHD

Endoscopy

If you need to examine internal organs or take a biopsy, you may need to do *una endocoscopia*, an endoscopy. Walk the patient through the procedures using the following phrases.

It is a procedure to examine internal organs.
Es un procedimiento para examinar los órganos internos.
ehs oon proh-seh-dee-mee-EHN-toh PAH-rah
eh-ksah-mee-NAHR lohs OHR-gah-nohs
een-TEHR-nohs

It is also used to take biopsies.
También se hace para tomar biopsias.
tahm-bee-EHN seh OO-sah PAH-rah
toh-MAHR bee-OP-see-ahs

A tube called an endoscope is introduced into the body.
Se introduce un tubo llamado endoscopio en el cuerpo.
seh een-troh-DOO-seh oon TOO-boh yah-MAH-doh
ehn-dohs-COH-pee-oh ehn ehl KWER-poh

To explain the different ways in which *un endoscopio*, an endoscope, can be introduced into the body, use *Se puede introducir* . . . (seh poo-EH-deh een-troh-doo-SEER)—it can be introduced . . .—followed by *por la boca* (pohr lah BOH-cah), through the mouth; *por un orificio natural* (pohr oon oh-ree-fee-SEE-oh nah-too-rahl), through an orifice; or *con una incisión quirúrgica* (OO-nah een-see-see-OHN kee-ROOR-hee-cah), through a surgical incision.

Bronchoscopy

When you need to examine *los bronquios* (lohs BROHN-kee-ohs), bronchi, you may have to perform *una broncoscopia* (OO-nah bron-cohs-COH-pee-ah).

A bronchoscopy is a procedure to see inside people's airways, or bronchi.
Una broncoscopia es un procedimiento para ver dentro de los bronquios.
OO-nah bron-cohs-COH-pee-ah ehs un proh-seh-dee-mee-EHN-toh PAH-rah vehr DEHN-troh deh lohs BRON-kee-ohs.

I am going to insert this tube in your mouth/nostril.
Voy a meter este tubo por su boca/foso nasal.
vohy ah meh-TEHR EHS-teh TOO-boh pohr soo BOH-cah/FOH-soh nah-SAHL

I am going to give you some medicine to help you relax.
Le voy a dar medicina para que se relaje.
leh vohy ah dahr me-dee-SEE-nah PAH-rah keh seh reh-LAH-heh

The nurse is going to insert an IV.
El/la enfermero/a le va a poner una sonda.
ehl/lah ehn-fehr-MEH-roh/rah leh vah ah poh-NEHR OO-nah SOHN-dah

The nurse is going to give you oxygen.
El/la enfermero/a le va a dar oxígeno.
ehl/lah ehn-fehr-MEH-roh/rah leh vah ah dahr
oh-KSEE-heh-noh

Put this mouthpiece in your mouth.
Póngase esta boquilla en la boca.
POHN-gah-seh EHS-tah boh-KEE-yah ehn lah BOH-cah

We are going to inject/spray anesthesia.
*Le vamos a dar anestesia con una inyección/con
un spray.*
leh VAH-mohs ah dahr ah-nehs-TEH-see-ah cohn
OO-nah een-yehk-see-OHN/cohn oon ehs-PRAH-ee.

Don't talk during this procedure.
No hable durante el test.
noh AH-bleh doo-RAHN-teh ehl test

Now that you have learned about different tests and
procedures and are able to share the results, you are ready
to learn how to discuss diagnoses and treatment options
in the next chapter.

Chapter 6
Diagnosis and Medications

You have now learned about the symptoms and performed the necessary tests. It is time to give a diagnosis and present possible treatments. This is a crucial part of your job, and this chapter will help you ensure that you present diagnosis and treatment options in a clear and efficient way.

Describing Conditions and Illnesses

There are endless conditions and illnesses that you can come across as a medical professional. Some are more common than others. Here is a list of some of the most common ones:

MEDICAL CONDITIONS AND ILLNESSES

anemia	*la anemia*
	lah ah-NEH-mee-ah
arthritis	*el artritis*
	ehl ahr-TREE-tees
asthma	*el asma*
	el AHS-mah
bronchitis	*la bronquitis*
	lah brohn-KEE-tees
cancer	*el cáncer*
	ehl CAHN-sehr
diabetes	*la diabetes*
	lah dee-ah-BEH-tehs
food poisoning	*la intoxicación alimentaria*
	lah een-toh-ksee-kah-see-OHN
	ah-lee-mehn-TAH-ree-ah
gastroenteritis	*la gastrointeritis*
	lah gahs-troh-een-teh-REE-tees
glaucoma	*el glaucoma*
	ehl glah-oo-COH-mah
gout	*la gota*
	lah GOH-tah
hepatitis	*la hepatitis*
	lah eh-pah-TEE-tees

MEDICAL CONDITIONS AND ILLNESSES—*continued*

high/low . . . .*la presión/tensión sanguínea alta/baja*
blood pressure   lah preh-see-OHN/tehn-see-OHN
                  sahn-GHEE-neh-ah AHL-tah/BAH-hah

high/low . . . .*el colesterol alto/bajo*
cholesterol   ehl coh-lehs-teh-ROHL
                  AHL-toh/BAH-hoh

hernia . . . .*la hernia*
                  lah EHR-nee-ah

hypertension . . . . . .*la hipertensión*
                  lah ee-pehr-tehn-see-OHN

hypoglycemia . . . . .*la hipoglicemia*
                  lah ee-poh-gloo-SEH-mee-ah

influenza, flu . . . . . .*la gripe*
                  lah GREE-peh

kidney stones . . . . .*las piedras en el riñón*
                  lahs pee-EH-drahs ehn ehl ree-NYON

laryngitis . . . .*la laringitis*
                  lah lah-reen-HEE-tees

leukemia . . . .*la leucemia*
                  lah leh-oo-SEH-mee-ah

lupus . . . .*el lupus*
                  ehl LOO-poos

meningitis . . . .*la meningitis*
                  lah meh-neen-HEE-tees

mumps . . . .*la parotiditis*
                  lah pah-roh-DEE-tees

osteoporosis . . . . . .*la osteoporosis*
                  lah ohs-teh-oh-poh-ROH-sees

MEDICAL CONDITIONS AND ILLNESSES—*continued*

Parkinson's disease	*la enfermedad de Parkinson, el Parkinsons* lah ehn-fehr-meh-DAHD deh PAHR-keen-sohn, ehl PAHR-keen-sohns
pneumonia	*la neumonía* lah neh-oo-moh-NEE-ah
polio	*el polio* ehl POH-lee-oh
ringworm	*la tiña* lah TEE-nyah
scarlet fever	*la escarlatina* lah ehs-cahr-lah-TEE-nah
sinusitis	*la sinusitis* lah see-noo-SEE-tees
tachycardia	*la taquicardia* lah tah-kee-CAHR-dee-ah
thyroid disease	*la enfermedad de tiroides* lah ehn-fehr-meh-DAHD deh tee-ROH-ee-dehs
tuberculosis	*la tuberculosis* lah too-behr-coo-LOH-sees
ulcer	*la úlcera* lah OOL-seh-rah

Giving a Diagnosis

To give a diagnosis, you can use the verb *tener* (to have). Say *Tiene usted . . .* followed by the condition. Note that the following sentences do not include the article *el/la* before the noun that describes the condition.

You have diabetes.
Tiene usted diabetes.
tee-EH-neh oos-TEHD dee-ah-BEH-tehs

You have hepatitis B.
Tiene usted hepatitis B.
tee-EH-neh oos-TEHD eh-pah-TEE-tees beh

Maria has epilepsy.
María tiene epilepsia.
mah-REE-ah tee-EH-neh eh-pee-LEHP-see-ah

 Fact

According to the OHM, the *Oficina de Salud de las Minorías*, leading causes of illness and death among Hispanics are *las enfermedades del corazón*, heart disease; *cáncer*, cancer; *accidentes*, accidents; *derrames,* stroke; and *diabetes*, diabetes. Other common conditions include *asma*, asthma; *enfermedades pulmonares obstructivas crónicas*, COPD; *VIH/SIDA*, HIV/AIDS; *obesidad*, obesity; and *tuberculosis*, tuberculosis.

Some conditions may require the infinitive article *un* or *una.*

You have an ulcer.
Tiene usted una úlcera.
tee-EH-neh oos-TEHD OO-nah OOL-seh-rah

Some patients may not be familiar with the specific diseases and you may have to explain what they are. Remember that nouns and adjectives agree in gender.

It is a malignant/benign tumor.
Es un tumor maligno/benigno.
eh soon too-MOHR mah-LEEG-noh/beh-NEEG-noh

To specify where the infection is, use *la infección de* . . . followed by the organ or body part.

It is an ear infection.
Es una infección del oído.
ehs OO-nah een-fek-see-OHN dehl oh-EE-doh

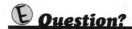 *Question?*

How can I reassure the patient?
If it is not a serious condition, you can say *No es muy serio* (noh ehs moo-EE SEH-ree-oh) or *Es muy común* (ehs moo-EE coh-MOON) for "it's common." If it is a serious condition, you can tell the patient not to worry and explain that there are effective treatments using *No se preocupe. Hay tratamientos efectivos.* (noh seh preh-oh-COO-peh. ahy trah-tah-mee-EHN-tohs eh-fek-TEE-vohs).

Treatment Options

There are usually different options for *tratamientos* (trah-tah-mee-EHN-tohs), treatments, of illnesses and conditions. It is important that the patient be aware of these options in order to make an informed decision.

There are different treatment options.
Hay varias opciones de tratamientos.
AH-ee VAH-ree-ahs op-see-OH-nehs deh
trah-tah-mee-EHN-tohs

COMMON TREATMENT OPTIONS

alternative	*los tratamientos alternativos*
treatments	lohs trah-tah-mee-EHN-tohs
	ahl-tehr-nah-TEE-vohs
blood transfusion	*la transfusión de sangre*
	lah trahns-foo-see-OHN deh
	SAHN-greh
change in	*el cambio en el estilo de vida*
lifestyle	ehl CAHM-bee-oh ehn ehl
	ehs-TEE-loh deh VEE-dah
chemotherapy	*la quimoterapia*
	lah kee-moh-teh-RAH-pee-ah
drugs	*las drogas*
	lahs DROH-gahs
experimental	*el tratamiento experimental*
treatment	ehl trah-tah-mee-EHN-toh
	ex-peh-ree-mehn-TAHL
medication	*la medicación*
	la meh-dee-cah-see-OHN

COMMON TREATMENT OPTIONS—*continued*

medicine . . . . *la medicina*
         lah meh-dee-SEE-nah

natural remedies . . *los remedios naturales*
         lohs reh-MEH-dee-ohs
         nah-too-RAH-lehs

radiation therapy . *la terapia de radiación*
         lah teh-RAH-pee-ah deh
         rah-dee-ah-see-OHN

surgery . . . . *la operación, la cirugía*
         lah oh-peh-rah-see-OHN, lah
         see-roo-HEE-ah

transplant . . . . *el transplante*
         ehl trahns-PLAHN-teh

Alert!

There are several words to describe medications, such as *la medicación*, *la medicina*, *el medicamento*, and *la droga*. The term *droga*, drug, is more commonly used to describe illegal drugs.

Expressing Preferences

Patients may express preference with the verb *preferir* (to prefer).

I prefer natural remedies.
Prefiero los remedios naturales.

preh-fee-EH-roh lohs reh-MEH-
dee-ohs nah-too-RAH-lehs

I prefer surgery.
Prefiero una operación.
preh-fee-EH-roh OO-nah oh-peh-rah-see-OHN

To ask the patient's preference, you can use the following phrases. You can present different options with *o* (or).

What do you prefer?
¿Qué prefiere?
keh preh-fee-EH-reh

What do you prefer, chemotherapy or surgery?
¿Qué prefiere, quimoterapia o cirugía?
keh preh-fee-EH-reh kee-moh-teh-
RAH-pee-ah oh see-roo-HEE-ah

 Fact

Some patients may ask for your recommendations
by saying *¿Qué recomienda usted?* for "What do you
recommend?" To make a recommendation, use *Le
recomiendo . . .* followed by the item. For example,
Le recomiendo la cirugía (I recommend surgery).

Sometimes there is only one option.

The only treatment is a transplant.
El único tratamiento es un transplante.
ehl OO-nee-coh trah-tah-mee-EHN-
toh ehs oon trahns-PLAHN-teh

The only option is medication.
La única opción es medicación.
lah OO-nee-cah op-see-OHN ehs
meh-dee-cah-see-OHN

Most Common Medications

As you write *la receta* (lah reh-SEH-tah), the prescription,
you may want to explain what type of medication you are
prescribing. Use these phrases:

Here is prescription for an antibiotic.
Aquí tiene una receta para un antibiótico.
ah-KEE tee-EH-neh OO-nah reh-SEH-tah
PAH-rah oon ahn-tee-bee-OH-tee-coh

This medicine is an antifungal.
Esta medicina es un antifúngico.
EHS-tah meh-dee-SEE-nah ehs oon
ahn-tee-FOON-geeh-coh

It is a cough suppressant.
Es un supresor de tos.
ehs oon soo-preh-SOHR deh tohs

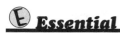 *Essential*

Medicines may be available *sin receta médica* (seen reh-SEH-tah MEH-dee-cah), over the counter, or you may need *una receta médica*, a prescription. The FDA website, *www.fda.gov*, offers a brochure in Spanish to help patients choose the best OTC medicine for you.

COMMON TYPES OF MEDICATION

analgesic	*el analgésico*
	ehl ah-nahl-HEH-see-coh
antacid	*el antiácido*
	ehl ahn-tee-AH-see-doh
antiarrhythmic	*la medicina antiarrítmica*
	lah meh-dee-SEE-nah ahn-tee-RREET-mee-cah
antibiotic	*el antibiótico*
	ehl ahn-tee-bee-OH-tee-coh
anticoagulant	*el anticoagulante*
	chl ahn-tee-coh-ah-goo-LAHN-teh
antidiarrheal	*el antidiarréico*
	ehl ahn-tee-dee-ah-RREH-ee-coh
anti-emetics	*el antiemético*
	ehl ahn-tee-eh-MEH-tee-coh
antifungal	*el antifúngico*
	ehl ahn-tee-FOON-hee-coh
antihypertensive	*el antihipertensivo*
	ehl ahn-tee-ee-pehr-tehn-SEE-voh

COMMON TYPES OF MEDICATION—*continued*

anti-inflammatory	*el antiinflamatorio*
	ehl ahn-tee-een-flah-mah-TOH-ree-oh
antineoplastic	*el antineoplásico*
	ehl ahn-tee-neh-oh-PLAH-see-coh
antipyretic	*el antipirético*
	ehl ahn-tee-pee-REH-tee-coh
antiviral	*la medicina antiviral*
	lah meh-dee-SEE-nah
	ahn-tee-vee-RAHL
aspirin	*la aspirina*
	lah ahs-pee-REE-nah
barbiturate	*el barbitúrico*
	ehl bahr-bee-TOO-ree-coh
cough suppressant	*el supresor de tos*
	ehl soo-preh-SOHR deh tohs
decongestant	*el descongestionante*
	ehl dehs-cohn-hehs-tee-oh-NAHN-teh
hormone	*la hormona*
	lah ohr-MOH-nah
ibuprofen	*el ibuprofeno*
	ehl eeh-boo-proh-FEH-noh
immuno-suppressant	*el inmunosupresor*
	ehl een-moo-noh-soo-preh-SOHR
morphine	*la morfina*
	lah morh-FEE-nah
muscle relaxant	*el relajante de músculos*
	ehl reh-lah-HAHN-teh deh
	MOOS-coo-lohs

COMMON TYPES OF MEDICATION—*continued*

vitamin . . . .*la vitamina*

lah vee-tah-MEE-nah

Instructions for Using Medications

As you prescribe medication, may also want to explain what form the medication comes in, and whether it needs to be taken orally or in any other form. Use *es . . .* (it is . . .) for singular and *son . . .* (They are . . .) for plural.

They are tablets.
Son unas pastillas.
sohn OO-nahs pahs-TEE-yahs

You need to take them orally/by mouth.
Tiene que tomarlas oralmente/por la boca.
tee-EH-neh keh toh-MAHR-lahs oh-rahl-MEHN-teh/
pohr lah BOH-cah

It is a gel.
Es una crema/un gel.
ehs OO-nah CREH-mah/oon hehl

You need to apply it in the affected area.
Tiene que aplicarlo en el área afectada.
tee-EH-neh keh ah-plee-CAHR-loh ehn
ehl AH-reh-ah ah-fec-TAH-dah

They are drops.
Son unas gotas.
sohn OO-nahs GOH-tahs

TYPES OF MEDICATIONS

chewtab . . . .*la tableta masticable*
    lah tah-BLEH-tah mahs-tee-CAH-bleh

cleanser. . . . .*el limpiador*
    ehl leem-pee-ah-DOHR

drops . . . .*las gotas*
    lahs GOH-tahs

gel . . . .*la crema, el gel*
    lah CREH-mah, ehl hehl

gel capsule . . . .*la cápsula de gel*
    lah CAP-soo-lah deh hehl

inhaler. . . . .*el inhalador*
    ehl een-ah-lah-DOHR

injection . . . .*la inyección*
    lah een-yek-see-OHN

ointment . . . .*el ungüento*
    eh loon-goo-EHN-toh

pill . . . .*la píldora, la pastilla*
    la PEEL-doh-rah, lah pahs-TEE-yah

nasal spray . . . .*el aerosol, el spray*
    ehl ah-eh-roh-SOHL, ehl SPRAH-ee

tablet . . . .*la pastilla*
    lah pahs-TEE-yah

Here some common uses of medications:

USES

to apply . . . . *aplicar*
ah-plee-CAHR

to attach . . . . *pegar*
peh-GAHR

to chew . . . . *masticar*
mahs-tee-CAHR

to insert . . . . *meter*
meh-TEHR

to put . . . . *poner*
po-NEHR

to spray . . . . *rociar*
roh-see-AHR

to take . . . . *tomar*
toh-MAHR

 Question?

How do I check whether the patient is taking other medications?
Every time you prescribe a medication or natural remedy, ask *¿Está tomando otras medicinas?* (ehs-TAH toh-MAHN-doh OH-trahs meh-dee-SEE-nahs), for "Are you taking any other medications?" Drug interactions may make your drug less effective and may cause side effects or serious health risks.

To explain the frequency of which the medication needs to be taken, you can use *cada . . . horas* (CAH-dah

. . . OH-rahs), for "every . . . hours," or . . . *veces al día* (VEH-sehs ahl DEE-ah), for " . . . times per day."

Take one every four hours.
Tome uno/a cada cuatro horas.
TOH-meh OO-noh CAH-dah KWAH-troh OH-rahs

Take two every six to eight hours.
Tome dos cada seis a ocho horas.
TOH-meh dohs CAH-dah seys ah OH-choh OH-rahs

Take one three times a day.
Tome una tres veces al día.
TOH-meh OO-nah trehs VEH-sehs ahl DEE-ah

Alert!

When giving instructions on how often a patient should take a medication, be particularly careful with using the word "once" in English. The same word in Spanish means "eleven." Even though it is pronounced differently—OHN-seh—it may create confusion. "Once" in Spanish is *una vez* (OO-nah vehs).

Take up to eight a day, as needed.
Tome hasta ocho por día, según sea necesario.
TOH-meh AHS-tah OH-choh pohr DEE-ah
seh-GOON SEH-ah neh-seh-SAH-ree-oh

Do not take more than six in twenty-four hours.
No tome más de seis en veinticuatro horas.
noh TOH-meh mahs deh seys ehn veh-een-tee-
KWAH-troh OH-rahs

Explaining Side Effects

Prepare the patient about possible *efectos secundarios*
(eh-FEHK-tohs seh-coon-DAH-ree-ohs), side effects, using
these phrases.

Some side effects are nausea and diarrhea.
*Algunos de los efectos secundarios son náusea
y diarrea.*
ahl-GOO-nohs deh lohs eh-FEHK-tohs seh-coon-DAH-
ree-ohs soh NAH-oo-seh-ah ee dee-ah-RREH-ah

Most people feel no side effects.
La mayoría de la gente no siente efectos secundarios.
lah mah-yoh-REE-ah deh lah HEHN-teh noh see-
EHN-teh eh-FEHK-tohs seh-coon-DAH-ree-ohs

You may lose your hair.
Es posible que pierda el cabello.
ehs poh-SEE-bleh keh pee-EHR-dah ehl cah-BEH-yoh

Do not drive or operate a machine while on
this medication.
*No maneje o use máquinas cuando esté tomando
esta medicación.*

noh mah-NEH-heh oh OO-seh MAH-kee-nahs
KWAHN-doh ehs-TEH toh-MAHN-doh EHS-tah
meh-dee-cah-see-OHN

Do not drink alcohol while on this medication.
No tome alcohol cuando esté tomando esta medicación.
noh TOH-meh ahl-coh-OHL KWAHN-doh ehs-TEH
toh-MAHN-doh EHS-tah meh-dee-cah-see-OHN

 Essential

Do not leave the patient wondering. To ask if the patient
has any questions, you can say *¿Tiene alguna pregunta?* (tee-EH-neh ahl-GOO-nah preh-GOON-tah)

Today, more and more medications include instructions in Spanish. Encourage your patients to look for them
and read them.

It is possible that the instructions are in Spanish.
Read them!
*Es posible que las instrucciones estén en español.
¡Léalas!*
ehs poh-SEE-bleh keh lahs eens-trook-see-OH-nehs
ehs-TEHN ehn ehs-pah-NYOHL. LEH-ah-lahs!

Chapter 7
Breaking the News

This chapter is about the best and worst parts of your job: sharing good and bad news. Patients will react very differently to life-changing situations. This may be more noticeable with people from cultures different from yours. Be ready for anything.

Surgery

In Spanish, surgery can be translated as *la operación* (la oh-peh-rah-see-OHN) or *la cirugía* (la see-roo-HEE-ah). Use the verb *necesitar*, which translates as "need," to explain the need of a surgery.

You need surgery.
Necesita usted cirugía/una operación.
neh-seh-SEE-tah oos-TEHD see-roo-HEE-ah/
OO-nah oh-peh-rah-see-OHN

To share the news to a relative, use *su* to express "your":

Your father needs an operation.
Su padre necesita una operación.
soo PAH-dreh neh-seh-SEE-tah OO-
nah oh-peh-rah-see-OHN

To explain the reasons for the surgery, you can use the verb *necesitar* followed by the verb that describes the reason.

We need to take a biopsy.
Necesitamos tomar una biopsia.
neh-seh-see-TAH-mohs toh-MAHR
OO-nah bee-OHP-see-ah

REASONS FOR SURGERY

explore the condition	*explorar la condición para*
to make a diagnosis	*diagnosticar*
	exploh-rahr lah cohn-dee-see-OHN
	PAH-rah dee-ag-nohs-tee-CAHR
remove diseased	*extirpar órganos o tejidos enfermos*
tissue or organs	ex-teer-PAHR OHR-gah-nohs oh
	teh-HEEH-dohs ehn-FEHR-mohs
restore proper	*reposicionar las estructuras a su*
function	*posición normal*
	reh-poh-see-see-oh-NAHR lahs
	ehs-trook-TOO-tahs ah soo
	poh-see-see-OHN nohr-MAHL
transplant tissue	*transplantar órganos o tejidos*
or organs	trahns-plahn-TAHR OHR-gah-nohs
	oh teh-HEEH-dohs
relieve pain	*aliviar el dolor*
	ah-lee-vee-AHR ehl doh-LOHR

You will find the names of different types of surgery and more information about them in Chapter 8.

Hospitalization

It is time to be admitted to *el hospital* (ehl ohs-pee-TAHL), the hospital. In Spanish, a need can be expressed with the verb *necesitar*, to need, or with the phrase *tener que*, which translates literally as "to have to."

You need to be hospitalized.
Necesita usted ser hospitalizado/a.
neh-seh-SEE-tah oos-TEHD sehr
ohs-pee-tah-lee-SAH-doh/dah

You have to stay at the hospital.
Tiene que quedarse en el hospital.
tee-eh-neh keh keh-DAHR-seh ehn ehl ohs-pee-TAHL

You will be in the hospital for ten days.
Estará en el hospital diez días.
ehs-tah-RAH ehn ehl ohs-pee-TAHL dee-EHS DEE-ahs

We need to monitor you for twenty-four hours.
Tenemos que observarle venticuatro horas.
teh-NEH-mohs keh obs-sehr-VAHR-leh
veyn-tee-KWAH-troh OH-rahs

We need to run some tests.
Tenemos que hacerle unos tests.
teh-NEH-mohs keh ah-SEHR-leh OO-nohs tests

You need hospital care.
Necesita usted cuidados de hospital.
neh-seh-SEE-tah oos-TEHD coo-ee-DAH-dohs
deh ohs-pee-TAHL

Alert!

There are several options in Spanish to describe places of healing. *El hospital* (ehl ohs-pee-TAHL) is used for "hospital" and *la clínica* (lah CLEE-nee-cah) is to refer to a smaller clinic. Another word to describe a place of healing, usually for terminal illness, is *el sanatorio* (sanatorium).

Discharge

"To discharge" is *dar de alta* (dahr deh AHL-tah). Share the *buenas noticias* (boo-EH-nahs noh-TEE-see-ahs), the good news, with these phrases:

We are going to discharge you.
Le vamos a dar de alta.
leh VAH-mohs ah dahr deh AHL-tah

You can go home today.
Se puede ir a casa hoy.
seh poo-EH-deh eer ah CAH-sah ohy

Patient Consent

There are several scenarios in which you will need to seek *el consentimiento del/de la paciente* (ehl cohn-sehn-tee-mee-EHN-toh dehl/deh lah pah-see-EHN-teh). Use these phrases:

We need your permission.
Necesitamos su permiso.
neh-seh-see-TAH-mohs soo pehr-MEE-soh

You need to sign a consent form.
Tiene que firmar un formulario de consentimiento.
tee-EH-neh keh feer-MAHR oon fohr-moo-LAH-
ree-oh deh cohn-sehn-tee-mee-EHN-toh

Use the preposition *para*, which in this context translates as "to," to explain the purpose of the permission.

Do we have permission to share this
information with . . . ?
*¿Nos da permiso para compartir esta
información con . . . ?*
nohs dah pehr-MEE-soh PAH-rah cohm-pahr-TEER
EHS-tah een-fohr-mah-see-OHN cohn . . .

Always try to explain what each form is. If your hospital or doctor's office offers forms in Spanish, make sure
you provide them.

Read and sign this Health Insurance Portability
and Accountability Act form (HIPAA).
*Lea y firme este Acta de Privacidad de
Información Médica.*
LEH-ah ee FEER-meh EHS-teh AHC-tah deh pree-vah-
see-DAHD deh een-fohr-mah-see-OHN MEH-dee-cah

REASONS FOR CONSENT FORMS

give a blood	.*hacer una transfusión de sangre*
transfusion	ah-SEHR OO-nah trahns-foo-see-OHN
	deh SAHN-greh
perform surgery . . .	.*operar*
	oh-peh-RAHR
perform a test	.*hacer un test*
	ah-SEHR oon test
use anesthesia	.*usar anestesia*
	oo-SAHR ah-nehs-TEH-see-ah
use a medication . .	.*usar una medicación*
	oo-SAHR OO-nah
	meh-dee-cah-see-OHN
use the patient's . . .	.*usar los órganos del/de la paciente*
organs	oo-SAHR lohs OHR-gah-nohs
	dehl/deh lah pah-see-EHN-teh
you can make	.*usted puede tomar las*
medical decisions	*decisiones médicas del paciente*
for the patient	oos-TEHD poo-EH-deh toh-MAHR
	lahs deh-see-see-OH-nehs
	MEH-dee-cahs dehl pah-see-EHN-teh
we cannot	.*no podemos mostrar su récord médico*
release your	noh poh-DEH-mohs mohs-TRAHR
medical records	soo REH-cohrd MEH-dee-coh

When the patient is *un/a menor de edad* (oon/OOH-nah meh-NOHR deh eh-DAHD), a minor, or if the patient is *incapacitado/a* (een-cah-pah-see-TAH-doh), incapacitated, you will need to ask for consent.

The patient (male/female) is a minor.
El/La paciente es menor de edad.
ehl/lah pah-see-EHN-teh ehs meh-
NOHR deh eh-DAHD

The patient is incapacitated.
El/La paciente está incapacitado/a.
ehl/lah pah-see-EHN-teh ehs-TAH
een-cah-pah-see-TAH-doh/dah

You need to make the decisions for him/her.
Usted tiene que tomar las decisiones por él/ella.
OOS-TEHD tee-EH-neh keh toh-MAHR lahs
deh-see-see-OH-nehs pohr ehl/EH-yah

Who is the legal health care agent?
¿Quién es el/la agente para el cuidado de la salud?
kee-EHN ehs ehl/lah ah-HEHN-teh PAH-rah
ehl coo-ee-DAH-doh deh lah sah-LOOD

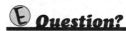

Question?

What do I say if the patient forgot to sign?
Ask whether he or she agrees with the document:
¿Está de acuerdo? (ehs-TAH deh ah-coo-EHR-
doh), for "Do you agree?" To remind the patient to
sign and date the form, say, *Por favor, firme aquí*,
for "please sign here" and *Escriba la fecha aquí* for
"write the date here."

At times, you will need to be informed of the patient's last wishes.

What are the patient's wishes?
¿Cuáles son los deseos del/de la paciente?
KWAH-lehs sohn lohs deh-SEH-ohs
dehl/deh lah pah-see-EHN-teh

Is there a do not resuscitate order?
¿Hay una orden de no resucitar?
ahy OO-nah OHR-dehn deh noh reh-soo-see-TAHR

Donating Organs

As a medical professional, you are aware of how important organ donation is for saving lives. You can use these phrases to recruit future donors. Be aware, however, that in some cultures organ donation is not accepted as it goes against religious beliefs.

Is the patient an organ donor?
¿Es el/la paciente donante de órganos?
ehs ehl/lah pah-see-EHN-teh doh-
NAHN-teh deh OHR-gah-nohs

Would you like to donate your organs?
¿Quiere usted donar sus órganos?
kee-EH-reh oos-TEHD doh-NAHR soos OHR-gah-nohs

Donating organs saves lives.
La donación de órganos salva vidas.
lah doh-nah-see-OHN deh OHR-gah-nohs
SAHL-vah VEE-dahs

You can choose which organs you want to donate.
Puede elegir qué órganos donar.
poo-EH-deh eh-leh-heer keh OHR-gah-nohs doh-NAHR

ORGANS AND TISSUE FOR DONATION

bone tissue	*los huesos*
	lohs oo-EH-sohs
cornea	*la córnea*
	lah COHR-neh-ah
eye	*el ojo*
	ehl OH-hoh
kidney	*el riñón*
	ehl ree-NYON
heart	*el corazón*
	ehl coh-rah-SOHN
heart valves	*las válvulas del corazón*
	lahs VAHL-voo-lahs dehl
	coh-rah-SOHN
intestines	*los intestinos*
	lohs een-tehs-TEE-nohs
ligaments	*los ligamentos*
	lohs lee-gah-MEHN-tohs
liver	*el hígado*
	ehl EE-gah-doh

ORGANS AND TISSUE FOR DONATION—*continued*

lung . . . . *.el pulmón*
ehl pool-MOHN

pancreas . . . . *.el páncreas*
ehl PAHN-kreh-ahs

skin tissue. . . . . . . *.la piel*
lah pee-EHL

stomach . . . . *.el estómago*
ehl ehs-TOH-mah-goh

tendons . . . . *.los tendones*
lohs tehn-DOH-nehs

vein . . . . *.la vena*
la VEH-nah

Death

Hopefully the following phrases will not be needed, but they will help you be prepared in case you have to announce the death of a patient to the family.

I am very sorry.
Lo siento mucho.
loh see-EHN-toh MOO-choh

There are several Spanish verbs to express death, such as *morir* (to die) and *fallecer* (to pass). In these types of situations, use *fallecer*.

The patient has passed away.
El/La paciente ha fallecido.
ehl/lah pah-see-EHN-teh ah fah-yeh-SEE-doh

When possible, explain the reasons of the outcome.

He/She did not respond well to the medications.
No respondió bien a la medicación.
noh rehs-pohn-dee-OH bee-EHN ah
lah meh-dee-cah-see-OHN

His/Her body did not accept the treatment.
Su cuerpo no aceptó el tratamiento.
soo KWEHR-poh noh ah-sehp-TOH
ehl trah-tah-mee-EHN-toh

It is always a good idea to refer patients to resources they can use to help them in difficult times.

We have counselors you can talk to.
Tenemos consejeros con los que puede hablar.
teh-NEH-mohs cohn-seh-HEH-rohs cohn
lohs keh poo-EH-deh ah-BLAHR

There are also online resources that patients can use. Medline Plus, the National Institute of Health's website, for instance, offers extensive resources in Spanish for people who have lost a loved one. Go to *www.nlm.nih.gov/medlineplus/spanish/bereavement.html*.

Sharing Life Expectancy

You may encounter patients who are facing *una enfermedad terminal* (OO-nah ehn-fehr-meh-DAHD tehr-mee-NAHL), a terminal illness.

I'm sorry. You have a terminal illness.
Lo siento. Tiene usted una enfermedad terminal.
loh see-EHN-toh. tee-EH-neh oos-TEHD OO-
nah ehn-fehr-meh-DAHD tehr-mee-NAHL

You have six months to live.
Le quedan seis meses de vida.
leh KEH dahn seys MEH-sehs deh VEE-dah

We can help you manage the pain.
Le podemos ayudar a controlar el dolor.
leh poh-DEH-mohs ah-yoo-DAHR ah
cohn-troh-lahr ehl doh-LOHR

Some issues are too serious to discuss with strong language barriers. This may be a good time to seek the help of a professional interpreter.

Please give me some time to find an
interpreter to explain the details.
*Por favor, permítame un poco de tiempo para
encontrar un intérprete que le explique los detalles.*
pohr fah-VOHR pehr-MEE-tah-meh oon
POH-coh deh tee-EHM-poh PAH-rah ehn-
cohn-TRAHR oon een-TEHR-preh-teh keh
leh eks-PLEE-keh lohs deh-TAH-yehs

Helping Patients Use Resources

There are several *recursos* (reh-COOR-sohs), resources, that can help you share information with patients, such as *páginas web* (PAH-hee-nahs web), websites; *líneas directas de teléfono* (LEE-neh-ahs dee-REHK-tahs deh teh-LEH-foh-noh), hotlines; and *folletos* (foh-YEH-tohs), brochures.

> You will find information at this website.
> *Encontrará información en esta página web.*
> ehn-cohn-trah-RAH een-fohr-mah-see-
> OHN ehn EHS-tah PAH-heeh-nah web

Sharing Phone Numbers

You can share a phone number by reading the digits individually. You can say *uno ochocientos* for 1-800.

> 1-800-222-1222
> *Uno ochocientos, dos, dos, dos, uno, dos, dos, dos.*
> OO-noh oh-choh-see-EHN-tohs dohs
> dohs dohs OO-noh dohs dohs dohs.

To explain what type of hotline it is, use *para*.

> It is a hotline for emergencies.
> *Es un teléfono para emergencias.*
> ehs oon teh-LEH-foh-noh deh eh-mehr-HEN-see-ahs

It is a poison control hotline.
Es un teléfono para el control de envenenamiento.
ehs oon teh-LEH-foh-noh PAH-rah ehl cohn-
TROHL deh ehn-veh-neh-nah-mee-EHN-toh

Reading Web Pages

To tell a patient to visit a particular website, use *vaya
a* (VAH-yah ah) followed by the name of the website.

Go to *www.mottep.org/espanol.*
Vaya a www.mottep.org/espanol.

When saying the name of the website, use *doble uve*
(DOH-bleh OO-veh) or *doble ve* (DOH-bleh veh) three
times to read "www". Use *punto* (POON-toh) for "dot" and
barra (BAH-rrah) for "slash."

www.aapcc.org
doble uve, doble uve, doble uve, a, a, p, c, c, punto, org
DOH-bleh OO-veh, DOH-bleh OO-veh, DOH-
bleh OO-veh ah ah peh seh seh POON-toh org

www.mottep.org/espanol
doble uve, doble uve, doble uve, m, o, t,
t, e, p, punto, org, barra, espanol
DOH-bleh OO-veh, DOH-bleh OO-veh, DOH-
bleh OO-veh EH-meh oh teh teh eh peh
POON-toh org BAH-rrah ehs-pah-nyohl

www.kidshealth.com
doble uve, doble uve, doble uve, kid-
shealth, punto, com
DOH-bleh OO-veh, DOH-bleh OO-veh, DOH-
bleh OO-veh kidshealth POON-toh com

 Essential

Some patients may not be familiar with the acronym FAQs, for "Frequently Asked Questions." When directing them to a website, encourage them to look at this section by explaining what it is: *Vaya a FAQ. Son las preguntas más frecuentes.* (VAH-yah ah EH-feh ah ko. sohn lahs preh-GOON-tahs mahs freh-koo-EHN-tehs).

To help patients find Spanish brochures on a particular website, use the following phrases.

Sharing Your Contact Information

Use the following phrases to share your *número de teléfono* (NOO-meh-roh deh teh-LEH-foh-noh), phone number, and your *email* (e-mail). Use *arroba* (ah-RROH-bah) for @.

My phone number is 212-555-3780
Mi número de teléfono es el dos, uno, dos, cinco, cinco, cinco, tres, siete, ocho, cero.

mee NOO-meh-roh deh teh-LEH-foh-noh ehs
ehl dohs OO-noh, dohs SEEN-coh SEEN-coh
SEEN-coh trehs see-EH-teh OH-choh SEH-roh

My e-mail is doc@dd.com
Mi email es doc, arroba, de, de, punto, com.
mee email ehs doc, ah-RROH-bah,
deh, deh, POON-toh com.

Chapter 8
Surgery

In Chapter 7, you learned how to break the news to a patient who needs surgery. Surgery can be intimidating, especially for patients who already bear the burden of navigating the system in a language they are unfamiliar with and a culture that is foreign to them. Whether you are dealing with major or minor surgery, your patients will need your guidance more than ever.

Types of Surgery

In Spanish, a doctor who performs a surgery is called *el/ la cirujano/a* (eh/lah see-roo-HAH-noh/nah). Surgeries can be *cirugía mayor* (see-roo-HEE-ah mah-YOHR), major surgery, or *cirugía menor* (see-roo-HEE-ah meh-NOHR), minor surgery.

Explaining Surgeries

To explain the nature of the surgery, use *Es una . . .* , "It is a . . . ," followed by the type of surgery. Note that *una*, a, takes the place of *la*, the.

It is a diagnostic surgery.
Es una cirugía diagnóstica.
ehs OO-nah see-roo-HEE-ah dee-ahg-NOHS-tee-cah

SURGERY TYPES

cosmetic surgery	*la cirugía cosmética* lah see-roo-HEE-ah cohs-MEH-tee-cah
curative surgery	*la cirugía curativa* lah see-roo-HEE-ah coo-rah-TEE-vah
diagnostic surgery	*la cirugía diagnóstica* lah see-roo-HEE-ah dee-ag-NOHS-tee-cah
elective surgery	*la cirugía opcional* lah see-roo-HEE-ah op-see-oh-NAHL
emergency surgery	*la cirugía de emergencia* lah see-roo-HEE-ah deh eh-mehr-HEHN-see-ah

SURGERY TYPES—*continued*

laparoscopic . . . . . . *la laparoscopia*
surgery   lah lah-pah-rohs-COH-pee-ah

laser surgery . . . . . . *la operación de láser*
     lah oh-peh-rah-see-OHN deh LAH-sehr

major surgery . . . . . *la cirugía mayor*
     lah see-roo-HEE-ah mah-YOHR

microsurgery . . . . . *la microcirugía*
     la mee-croh-see-roo-HEE-ah

minor surgery . . . . . *la cirugía menor*
     lah see-roo-HEE-ah meh-NOHR

palliative . . . . *la cirugía paliativa*
surgery   lah see-roo-HEE-ah pah-lee-ah-TEE-vah

plastic surgery . . . *la cirugía plástica*
     lah see-roo-HEE-ah PLAHS-tee-cah

preventive . . . . *la cirugía preventiva*
surgery   lah see-roo-HEE-ah pre-vehn-TEE-vah

required surgery . . *la cirugía requerida*
     lah see-roo-HEE-ah reh-keh-REE-dah

You can specify the type of surgery needed by using *la operación de* followed by the body part or organ to be operated on. *La operación de la espalda*, for instance, is back surgery. When the body part is a masculine noun that takes *el*, use *del* (*de + el*). For example, *la operación del corazón* (heart surgery). Here are the names of some common operations:

SURGERIES

brain surgery	*la operación del cerebro*
	lah oh-peh-rah-see-OHN dehl
	seh-REH-broh
bypass heart	*la cirugía de derivación cardíaca*
surgery	lah see-roo-HEE-ah deh deh-ree-
	vah-see-OHN cahr-dee-AH-cah
cervical spine . . .	*la cirugía de la columna cervical*
surgery	lah see-roo-HEE-ah deh lah
	coh-LOOM-nah sehr-vee-CAHL
gall bladder	*la operación de la vesicula biliar*
surgery	lah oh-peh-rah-see-OHN deh lah
	veh-SEE-coo-lah bee-lee-AHR
hip replacement . .	*la operación de la cadera*
surgery	lah oh-peh-rah-see-OHN deh lah
	cah-DEH-rah
lung surgery	*la cirugía de pulmón*
	lah see-roo-HEE-ah de pool-MOHN
open-heart	*la operación de corazón abierto*
surgery	lah oh-peh-rah-see-OHN deh
	coh-rah-SOHN ah-bee-EHR-toh
small intestine . . .	*la operación de extirpación del*
removal surgery	*intestino delgado*
	lah oh-peh-rah-see-OHN deh
	ex-teer-pah-see-OHN dehl een-tehs-
	TEE-noh dehl-GAH-doh
stomach surgery. . .	*la operación del estómago*
	lah oh-peh-rah-see-OHN dehl
	ehs-TOH-mah-goh

Explaining Anesthesia Options

Part of the process is to let patients know about the anesthesia they will be getting, as well as to collect the patient's history regarding this matter. The following phrases will help you accomplish this:

Is this your first surgery?
¿Es esta su primera operación?
ehs EHS-tah soo pree-MEH-rah oh-peh-rah-see-OHN

Have you had anesthesia before?
¿Ha recibido anestesia antes?
ah reh-see-BEE-doh ah-nehs-TEH-see-ah AHN-tehs

You will be getting local anesthesia.
Recibirá usted anestesia local.
reh-see-bee-RAH oos-TEHD ah-nehs-TEH-see-ah loh-CAHL

ANESTHESIA TYPES

anesthesia	*la anestesia general/total*
	lah ah-nehs-TEH-see-ah
	heh-neh-RAHL toh-TAHL
conscious or	*la sedación consciente* or *intravenosa*
intravenous	lah seh-dah-see-OHN cohns-see-
sedation	EHN-teh/een-trah-veh-NOH-sah
local anesthesia . . .	*la anestesia local*
	lah ah-nehs-TEH-see-ah loh-CAHL

ANESTHESIA TYPES—*continued*

regional . . . . *la anestesia regional or parcial*
anesthesia   lah ah-nehs-TEH-see-ah reh-hee-
oh-NAHL/pahr-see-AHL

epidural . . . . *la anestesia epidural*
lah ah-nehs-TEH-see-ah
eh-pee-doo-RAHL

Comparing Surgery to Other Treatments

Patients may have questions about upcoming surgery, and you may find yourself comparing them to other treatments. To compare two items in Spanish, use *más*, followed by the adjective and *que*. For instance, *más efectiva que . . .* translates as "more effective than."

This surgery is more effective than only medication.
Esta operación es más efectiva que sólo medicación.
EHS-tah oh-peh-rah-see-OHN ehs mahs eh-fehk-TEE-vah keh SOH-loh meh-dee-cah-see-OHN

This surgery is more effective than physical therapy.
Esta operación es más efectiva que la terapia física.
EHS-tah oh-peh-rah-see-OHN ehs mahs eh-fehk-TEE-vah keh lah teh-RAH-pee-ah FEE-see-cah

To express that one item is less of something than another, use *menos* + adjective + *que*. For instance, *menos efectiva que . . .* translates as "less effective than."

Physical therapy is less effective than this surgery.
La terapia física es menos efectiva que esta operación.
lah teh-RAH-pee-ah ehs MEH-nohs eh-fehk-
TEE-vah keh EHS-tah oh-peh-rah-see-OHN

The recovery of this surgery is less painful.
La recuperación de esta operación es menos dolorosa.
lah reh-coo-peh-rah-see-OHN deh EHS-tah oh-peh-
rah-see-OHN ehs MEH-nohs doh-loh-ROH-sah

ⓔ *Alert!*

In Spanish, comparisons are always made with *más
. . . que* (more . . . than) and *menos . . . que* (less
. . . than). In English, adjectives sometimes change
form, as in long/longer. In Spanish, the adjective
remains unchanged.

When surgery is la *única opción* (lah OO-nee-cah op-
see-OHN), the only option, you can say:

This surgery is the only way to fix the problem.
*Esta operación es la única manera de solucionar
el problema.*
EHS-tah oh-peh-rah-see-OHN ehs lah OO-nee-cah
mah-NEH-rah deh soh-loo-see-oh-NAHR ehl
proh-BLEH-mah

This surgery could lead to a better quality of life.
*Esta operación le puede ofrecer una calidad
de vida mejor.*
EHS-tah oh-peh-rah-see-OHN leh poo-EH-deh
oh-freh-SEHR OO-nah cah-lee-DAHD deh VEE-dah
meh-HOHR

Preparing for Surgery

Use these phrases to get the patient ready before going to
la sala de operaciones (lah SAH-lah deh oh-peh-rah-see-
OH-nehs), the operating room.

Don't drink after midnight.
No beba después de la medianoche.
noh BEH-bah dehs-poo-EHS deh lah
meh-dee-ah-NOH-cheh

Don't eat the day of the surgery.
No coma el día de la operación.
noh COH-mah ehl DEE-ah deh lah
oh-peh-rah-see-OHN

Take an enema to empty the bowels.
Póngase un enema para vacíar el intestino.
POHN-gah-seh oon eh-NEH-mah PAH-rah
vah-see-AHR ehl een-tehs-TEE-noh

There are certain items that patients should not have the day of surgery, such as *el maquillaje* (ehl mah-kee-YAH-heh), makeup; *las lentes de contacto* (lahs LEHN-tehs deh conTAHC-toh), contact lenses; *las joyas* (lahs HOH-yahs), jewelry; and *los objetos de valor* (lohs ob-HEH-tohs deh vah-LOHR), valuables. To ask a patient not to bring something use *No traiga . . .* , "Do not bring" . . . , followed by the noun without the article *el, la, los*, or *las*.

Do not bring any valuables.
No traiga objetos de valor.
noh trah-EE-gah ob-HEH-tohs deh vah-LOHR

You cannot wear your dentures.
No puede llevar la dentadura postiza.
noh poo-EH-deh yeh-VAHR lah dehn-tah-DOO-rah pohs-TEE-sah

You can further prepare the patient with these phrases:

Please wear this identification bracelet.
Por favor póngase esta pulsera de identificación.
pohr fah-VOHR POHN-gah-seh EHS-tah pool-SEH-rah deh ee-dehn-tee-fee-cah-see-OHN

We will shave the area of operation.
Vamos a afeitar el área de la operación.
VAH-mohs ah ah-feh-ee-TAHR ehl AH-reh-ah deh lah oh-peh-rah-see-OHN

The operation will last two hours.
La operación durará dos horas.
lah oh-peh-rah-see-OHN doo-rah-RAH dohs OH-rahs

 Question?

What do I say if I want to comfort the patient?
Use the following reassuring words: *Todo saldrá bien* (TOH-doh sahl-DRAH bee-EHN) for "everything will be okay" and *No sentirá usted dolor* (noh sehn-tee-RAH oos-TEHD doh-LOHR) for "you won't feel any pain."

We need to move you to this gurney.
Tenemos que moverle a esta camilla.
teh-NEH-mohs keh moh-VEHR-
leh ah EHS-tah cah-MEE-yah

We are going to take you to the operating room.
Vamos a llevarle a la sala de operaciones.
VAH-mohs ah yeh-VAHR-leh ah lah SAH-
lah deh oh-peh-rah-see-OH-nehs

Prognosis and Recovery
Let's start by sharing the good news of a successful surgery.

The surgery went very well.
La operación fue muy bien.
lah oh-peh-rah-see-OHN foo-EH moo-EEY bee-EHN

Once the surgery is completed, the patient will be transferred to *la sala de recuperación* (SAH-lah deh reh-coo-peh-rah-see-OHN), the recovery room. Use *Vamos a . . .* (VAH-mohs ah), we are going to, followed by the following actions to prepare patients for what is to come.

CLINICAL STAFF ACTIONS

check lines, ...	*revisar las líneas, tubos o drenajes*
tubes, or drains	reh-vee-SAHR lahs LEE-neh-ahs TOO-bohs oh dreh-NAH-hehs
check the	*revisar la herida*
wound	reh-vee-SAHR lah EH-ree-dah
monitor vital	*monitorizar los signos vitales*
signs	moh-nee-toh-ree-SAHR lohs SEEG-nohs vee-TAH-lehs
monitor for any	*monitorizar cualquier tipo de complicación*
signs of	
complications	moh-nee-toh-ree-SAHR coo-ahl-kee-EHR TEE-poh deh cohm-plee-cah-see-OHN
monitor the	*monitorizar el nivel de conciencia*
level of	moh-nee-toh-ree-SAHR ehl nee-VEHL
conciousness	deh cohn-see-EHN-see-ah
take the	*tomar la temperatura*
temperature	toh-MAHR lah tehm-peh-rah-TOO-rah

Here are some further questions to ask the patient:

Are you in any pain?
¿Siente usted dolor?
see-EHN-teh oos-TEHD doh-LOHR

What did you drink today?
¿Qué bebió usted hoy?
keh beh-bee-OH oos-TEHD OH-ee

The length of time spent in recovery depends on the type of surgery performed. A patient can in some cases aid the speed of the recovery by doing certain exercises. To suggest exercises your patient should do use *Debe . . .* (DEH-beh), which translates as "you should."

You should change positions.
Debe cambiar de posición.
DEH-beh cahm-bee-AHR deh poh-see-see-OHN

It is important that the patient does not feel forced to do something he or she is not able to do.

Do it only if you can.
Hágalo sólo si puede.
AH-gah-loh SOH-loh see poo-EH-deh

Here are some further instructions for patients who go home after surgery:

Keep your wound dry and clean for
the first twenty-four hours.
*Mantenga la herida seca y limpia durante
las primeras veinticuatro horas.*
mahn-TEHN-gah lah eh-REE-dah SEH-cah
ee LEE-pee-ah doo-RAHN-teh lahs pree-
MEH-rahs veyn-tee-KWAH-troh OH-rahs

If it continues to bleed, call us.
Si sigue sangrando, llámenos.
see SEE-gueh sahn-GRAHN-doh YAH-meh-nohs

We do not need to remove your stitches.
No tenemos que remover los puntos.
noh teh-NEH-mohs keh reh-moh-
VEHR lohs POON-tohs

 Question?

**Will my American accent get in the way when
trying to give crucial information?**
The key is to get those vowels right! Remember that
a is always pronounced "ah," *e* is "eh," *i* is "ee," *o*
is "oh," and *u* is "oo." Is you master these, you will
sound more like a native speaker. However, if you
feel you are not being understood, write down the
words or use visuals. Some information is too important to be lost in translation.

Your body will absorb the stitches.
Su cuerpo absorberá los puntos.
soo KWEHR-poh ab-sohr-beh-RAH lohs POON-tohs

You need to come so we can
remove your stitches/staples.
*Tiene que venir para que le quite-
mos los puntos/las grapas.*
tee-EH-neh keh veh-NEER PAH-rah keh leh kee-
TEH-mohs lohs POON-tohs/lahs GRAH-pahs

Remove the bandages in two days.
Quítese las vendas en dos días.
KEE-teh-seh lahs VEHN-dahs ehn dohs DEE-ahs

Your scar may be red. This is normal.
La cicatriz puede estar roja. Es normal.
lah see-cah-TREES poo-EH-deh ehs-
TAHR ROH-hah. ehs nohr-MAHL

Your throat may be sore for a day.
Es posible que le moleste la garganta un día.
ehs poh-SEE-bleh keh leh moh-LEHS-teh lah
gahr-GAHN-tah oon DEE-ah

Do not drive or make important decisions for
twenty-four hours after general anesthesia.
*No maneje o tome decisiones importantes las
primeras veinticuatro horas después de la
anestesia general.*

noh mah-NEH-heh oh TOH-meh deh-see-see-OH-
nehs eem-pohr-TAHN-tehs lahs pree-MEH-rahs
veyn-tee-KWAH-troh OH-rahs dehs-poo-EHS
deh lah ah-nehs-TEH-see-ah heh-neh-RAHL

Alert!

There are two ways to say "to drive" in Spanish:
manejar (mah-NEH-hahr), which is mostly used in
Latin America, and *conducir* (cohn-doo-SEER),
which is mostly used in Spain.

Call your doctor if you have vomiting, fever,
or signs of infection at the surgical site.
*Llame a su médico/a si tiene vómitos, fiebre o
signos de infección en el área de la operación.*
YAH-meh a soo MEH-dee-coh/cah see tee-
EH-neh VOH-mee-tohs, fee-EH-breh oh
SEEG-nohs de een-fehk-see-OHN ehn ehl
AH-reh-ah deh lah oh-peh-rah-see-OHN

Chapter 9
OB/GYN and Pediatrics

Your Spanish-speaking patients' culture may differ greatly from yours. This may be most evident when talking about matters of childrearing, personal choices, or sex. Remember to keep an open mind and offer as much information as you can. This chapter will help you navigate some of the situations you may encounter.

Common Problems and Treatments

Whether you are a *ginecólogo/a* (hee-neh-COH-loh-goh/gah), a gynecologist, or not, you may come across a female patient with some of these symptoms:

SYMPTOMS

abnormalities in the nipple	*las abnormalidades en el pezón* lahs ab-nohr-mah-lee-DAH-dehs ehn ehl peh-SOHN
breast pain	*el dolor de pecho/seno* ehl doh-LOHR deh PEH-choh/ SEH-noh
burning sensation	*el ardor* ehl ahr-DOHR
changes in menstruation	*los cambios en el periodo* lohs CAHM-bee-ohs ehn ehl peh-ree-OH-doh
excessive bleeding	*el sangrar excesivamente* ehl sahn-GRAHR ex-seh-see- vah-MEHN-teh
excessive weight gain/loss	*la subida/pérdida de peso excesiva* lah soo-BEE-dah/PEHR-dee-dah deh PEH-soh ex-seh-SEE-vah
heavy periods	*los periodos fuertes* lohs peh-ree-OH-dohs foo-EHR-tehs
hot flashes	*la sensación de calor intenso* lah sehn-sah-see-OHN deh cah-LOHR een-TEHN-soh
irritation	*la irritación* lah ee-rree-tah-see-OHN

SYMPTOMS—*continued*

itchiness	*el picor*
	ehl pee-COHR
lump	*el bulto*
	el BOOL-toh
mood swing	*el cambio de genio*
	ehl CAHM-bee-oh deh HEH-nee-oh
night sweats	*los sudores nocturnos*
	lohs soo-DOH-rehs nohc-TOOR-nohs
painful	*el dolor al orinar*
urination	ehl doh-LOHR ahl oh-ree-NAHR
spotting	*las manchas*
	lahs MAHN-chahs
strong cramps	*los calambres fuertes*
	lohs cah-LAHM-brehs foo-EHR-tehs
urinary	*la incontinencia*
incontinence	lah een-cohn-tee-NEHN-see-ah
vaginal	*las secreciones vaginales*
discharge	lahs seh-creh-see-OH-nehs
	vah-hee-NAH-lehs

To ask whether a patient has a particular symptom, you can use the verb *tener* (to have). Note that you do not need to add the article *el* or *la* in most cases.

Do you have strong cramps?
¿Tiene calambres fuertes?
tee-EH-neh cah-LAHM-brehs foo-EHR-tehs

Do you have vaginal discharge?
¿Tiene secreciones vaginales?
tee-EH-neh seh-creh-see-OH-nehs vah-hee-NAH-lehs

Getting to Know your Patient

In order to make the right diagnosis, you will need to know about the patient's social and medical history. Here are some general questions about *la menstruación*, menstruation, that will help you get started.

Do you still menstruate?
¿Menstrua usted todavía?
mehns-TROO-ah oos-TEHD toh-dah-VEE-ah

When was your last menstrual period?
¿Cuándo fue su último periodo?
KWAN-doh foo-EH soo OOL-tee-moh peh-ree-OH-doh

Are your periods regular?
¿Son regulares sus periodos?
sohn reg-goo-LAH-rehs soos peh-ree-OH-dos

How often do you get your period?
¿Cada cuánto tiene el periodo?
CAH-dah KWAN-toh tee-EH-neh ehl peh-ree-OH-doh

How long does your period last?
¿Cuánto le dura el periodo?
KWAN-toh leh DOO-rah ehl peh-ree-OH-doh

Describe your menstrual flow.
Describa su flujo menstrual.
dehs-CREE-bah soo FLOO-hoh mehns-troo-AHL

Do you have cramps?
¿Tiene usted calambres?
tee-EH-neh oss-TEHD cah-LAHM-brehs

Have you ever been pregnant?
¿Ha estado embarazada alguna vez?
ah ehs-TAH-doh ehm-bah-rah-SAH-dah
ahl-GOO-nah vehs

How many times?
¿Cuántas veces?
KWAN-tahs VEH-sehs

Is there a chance that you are pregnant now?
¿Hay posibilidad de que esté embarazada ahora?
ah-ee poh-see-bee-lee-DAHD deh keh ehs-TEH
ehm-bah-rah-SAH-dah ah-OH-rah

Are you sexually active?
¿Está teniendo relaciones sexuales?
ehs-TAH teh-nee-EHN-doh reh-lah-see-OH-nehs
seh-ksoo-AH-lehs

Describe the vaginal discharge.
Describa la secreción vaginal.
dehs-CREE-bah lahs seh-creh-see-OHN vah-hee-NAHL

Is it clear? Yellow? Brown?
¿Es transparente?¿Amarilla?¿Marrón?
ehs trahns-pah-REHN-teh, ah-mah-REE-yah,
mah-RROHN

 Question?

What do I do if my patient does not want to share personal information?
If you are a man, she may feel more comfortable talking to a female nurse or doctor. Ask *¿Prefiere hablar con una mujer?* (preh-fee-EH-reh ah-BLAHR cohn OO-nah moo-HEHR), for "Do you prefer to talk to a woman?". If she seems embarrassed, you can say, *Necesito esta información para ayudarla* (neh-seh-SEE-toh EHS-tah een-fohr-mah-see-OHN PAH-rah ah-yoo-DAHR-lah) to let her know you need information to help her.

Now that you have some basic information about the patient, you will need to examine her. The next sections will help you with some common exams.

Common Tests and Exams

Walking the patient through tests and procedures is particularly important when dealing with very sensitive areas. A pelvic exam definitely qualifies as one of these.

I am going to do a pelvic exam.
Voy a hacerle un examen pélvico.
vohy ah ah-SEHR-leh oon eh-
KSAH-mehn PEHL-vee-coh

I am going to put my fingers in your vagina.
Voy a meter mis dedos en su vagina.
vohy ah meh-TEHR mees DEH-
dohs ehn soo vah-HEE-nah

Relax. It will not hurt.
Relájese. No le va a doler.
reh-LAI I-heh-seh. noh leh vah ah doh-LEHR

I am going to insert this speculum into your vagina.
Voy a meter este espéculo en su vagina.
vohy ah meh-TEHR EHS-teh ehs-PEH-coo-loh

I need to examine your cervix.
Tengo que examinar su cérvix.
TEHN-goh keh eh-ksah-mee-NAHR soo SEHR-veex

It will feel a little cold.
Sentirá un poco de frío.
sehn-tee-RAH oon POH-coh deh FREE-oh

I am going to put my finger in your rectum.
Voy a poner mi dedo en su recto.
vohy ah poh-NEHR mee DEH-doh ehn soo REC-toh

Breast Exam

There are posters and other visual aids available that show women how to conduct a breast exam. If possible, display some in your place of work to show your non-English-speaking patients. Remember there are two ways to say breast: *pecho* (PEH-choh) and *seno* (SEH-noh).

I am going to examine your breasts.
Voy a examinar sus senos.
vohy ah eh-ksah-mee-NAHR soos SEH-nohs

Raise your arm.
Levante el brazo.
leh-VAHN-teh ehl BRAH-soh

Put your hand behind your head.
Ponga la mano detrás de la cabeza.
POHN-gah la MAH-noh deh-
TRAHS deh lah cah-BEH-sah

I am looking for lumps.
Busco a ver si hay algún bulto.
BOOS-coh ah vehr see ah-EE ahl-GOON BOOL-toh

You need to do a breast self-examination every month.
Debe hacer un auto-examen de sus senos cada mes.
DEH-beh ah-sehr oon ah-OO-toh eh-XAH-mehn
deh soos SEH-nohs CAH-dah mehs

Fact

Nearly 13 percent of all women will get *cáncer de pecho/seno/mama*, breast cancer, in their lifetime. Early detection through monthly breast self-exams and a yearly mammography after age forty offers the best chance of catching breast cancer early and beating the disease. Ninety-six percent of women who treat breast cancer early are cancer-free after five years.

You can get dressed now.
Ya puede vestirse.
yah poo-EH-deh vehs-TEER-seh

OB/GYN: Diagnosis

A diagnosis can be *buenas noticias* (boo-EH-nahs noh-TEE-see-ahs), good news, or *malas noticias* (MAH-lahs noh-TEE-see-ahs), bad news, for patients.

Sharing Test Results

Let's start with the good news first. Here are ways to share some test results:

Your Pap smear is negative.
Su prueba de Pap es negativa.
soo proo-EH-bah deh pahp ehs neh-gah-TEE-vah

Your pregnancy test is positive.
Su test de embarazo es positivo.
soo test deh ehm-bah-RAH-soh ehs poh-see-TEE-voh

When the results are inconclusive and you need more tests, say:

The results are inconclusive.
Los resultados no son concluyentes.
lohs reh-sool-TAH-dohs noh sohn
con-cloo-YEHN-tehs

We need to do more tests.
Tenemos que hacer más tests.
teh-NEH-mohs keh ah-SEHR mahs tests

If the tests came back negative, say:

I'm sorry. The test was negative.
Lo siento. El test salió negativo.
loh see-EHN-toh. ehl test sah-lee-OH neh-gah-TEE-voh

To give a diagnosis, you can use *Tiene usted . . . (You have . . .).*

You have a urinary tract infection.
Tiene usted una cistitis.
tee-EH-neh oss-TEHD OO-nah sees-TEE-tees

You have ovarian cancer.
Tiene usted cáncer ovárico.
tee-EH-neh oss-TEHD CAHN-sehr oh-VAH-ree-coh

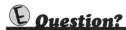 *Question?*

How do I reassure the patient if the news is not good?
One way is to tell her not to worry by saying *No se preocupe* (noh seh preh-oh-COO-peh), and explain that there are some effective treatments available, *Hay muchos tratamientos efectivos* (AH-ee MOO-chohs trah-tah-mee-EHN-tohs eh-fehk-TEE-vohs). Have some literature available in Spanish for the patient to educate herself.

As you can see in the above examples, the article *el/la* is sometimes omitted. You will find it in parenthesis in the list of conditions below. Some conditions may take *un, una, unas,* or *unos.*

CONDITIONS

a urinary tract . . . . *una cistitis*
infection   OO-nah sees-TEE-tees
breast cancer . . . . . *(el) cáncer de pecho/seno*
          ehl CAHN-sehr deh PEH-choh/SEH-noh
cervical cancer . . . . *(el) cáncer cervical/cérvico*
          ehl CAHN-sehr sehr-vee-CAHL/
          SEHR-vee-coh

CONDITIONS—*continued*

cervical dysplasia. .*(la) displasia cervical*
lah dees-PLAH-see-ah sehr-vee-CAHL

ovarian cancer . . . .*(el) cáncer de ovario/ovárico*
CAHN-sehr deh oh-VAH-ree-oh/
oh-VAH-ree-coh

ovarian cysts. . . . . .*unos quistes en el ovario*
OO-nohs KEES-tehs ehn ehl
oh-VAH-ree-oh

uterine fibroids. . . .*el fibroma uterino*
ehl fee-BROH-mah oo-teh-REE-noh

a yeast infection. . .*una infección fúngica/(la) candidiasis*
OO-nah een-fek-see-OHN FOON-
heeh-cah/lah cahn-DEE-dee-ah-sees

 Fact

According to the American Cancer Society, one in
every three Hispanic women in the United States
will be diagnosed with cancer in her lifetime. The
most commonly diagnosed cancer among Hispanic
women is breast cancer. You can refer your Hispanic
clients to the American Cancer Society website in
Spanish (*www.cancer.org*) for information on the
topic.

Sexually Transmitted Diseases

Las enfermedades de transmisión sexual (lahs ehn-fehr-
meh-DAH-dehs deh trans-mee-see-OHN seh-ksoo-AHL),

STDs, affect both *los hombres* (lohs OHM-brehs), men, and *las mujeres* (lahs moo-HEH-rehs), women. In addition to the symptoms presented earlier in the chapter, patients may have the following symtoms.

SYMPTOMS

abdominal pain	*el dolor en el abdomen*
	ehl doh-LOHR ehn ehl ab-DOH-mehn
dripping	*el goteo*
	ehl goh-TEH-oh
blister	*la ampolla*
	lah ahm POH-yah
chills	*los escalofríos*
	lohs ehs-cah-loh-FREE-ohs
sores	*las llagas*
	lahs YAH-gahs
warts	*las verrugas*
	lahs veh-RROO-gahs

To check whether a patient has any of the above symptoms, use *¿Tiene . . . ?*

Do you have blisters?
¿Tiene ampollas?
tee-EH-neh ahm-POH-yahs

You will also need information about the patient's sexual history. "To have sexual intercourse" in Spanish is *tener relaciones sexuales* (teh-NEHR reh-lah-see-OH-ehs seh-ksoo-AH-lehs).

Have you had sexual contact with anyone?
¿Ha tenido contacto sexual con alguien?
ah teh-NEE-doh cohn-TAHC-toh seh-
ksoo-AHL cohn AHL-ghee-EHN

Was it with a woman or a man?
¿Fue con una mujer o un hombre?
foo-EH cohn OO-nah MOO-hehr oh oon OHM-breh

Did you have rectal or anal contact?
¿Tuvo contacto por el recto o ano?
TOO-voh cohn-TAHC-toh pohr ehl
REHC-toh oh ehl AH-noh

Again, to make a diagnosis you can use the verb *tener* (to have). Note that you do not need to add the article *el/la* before the name of the condition.

You have herpes.
Tiene usted herpes.
tee-EH-neh oos-TEHD EHR-pehs

STDS

AIDS	*(el) SIDA*
	ehl SEE-dah
chlamydia	*(la) clamidia*
	lah clah-MEE-dee-ah
gonorrhea	*(la) gonorrea*
	lah goh-noh-REEH-ah

STDS—*continued*

hepatitis B	*(la) hepatitis B*
	lah eh-pah-TEE-tees beh
herpes	*(el) herpes*
	ehl EHR-pehs
HIV	*(el) HIV*
	ehl AH-cheh ee veh
HPV	*una infección genital por VPH*
	OO-nah een-fehk-see-OHN heh-
	nee-TAHL pohr veh peh AH-cheh
pelvic	*(la) enfermedad inflamatoria pélvica*
inflammatory	lah ehn-fehr-meh-DAHD een-flah-
disease	mah-TOH-ree-ah PEHL-vee-cah
syphilis	*(la) sífilis*
	lah SEE-fee-lees

Pregnancy and Childbirth

Pregnancy is an exciting and intense time for a woman. Many women experience anxiety and will rely on their doctors for support. You efforts to communicate in Spanish will be greatly appreciated. Let's get started with some general vocabulary related to pregnancy and childbirth.

CHILDBIRTH AND PREGNANCY

abortion	*el aborto*
	ehl ah-BOHR-toh
to break water	*romper la bolsa de agua*
	rohm-PEHR lah BOHL-sah deh
	ah-GOO-aha

CHILDBIRTH AND PREGNANCY—*continued*

to breastfeed. . . . . .*dar el pecho, dar el seno, amamantar*
dahr ehl PEH-choh, dahr ehl
SEH-noh, ah-mah-mahn-TAHRå

cesarean . . . .*la operación cesárea*
section lah oh-peh-rah-see-OHN
seh-SAH-reh-ah

contraction . . . .*la contracción*
lah cohn-trahk-see-OHN

to deliver . . . .*dar a luz, parir*
dahr ah looz, pah-REER

delivery . . . .*el parto*
ehl PAHR-toh

episiotomy. . . . .*la episotomía*
lah eh-pee-see-oh-toh-MEE-ah

fallopian tubes . . . .*las trompas de falopio*
lahs TROHM-pahs deh
fah-LOH-pee-oh

labor pains . . . .*los dolores del parto*
lohs doh-LOH-rehs dehl PAHR-toh

miscarriage. . . . . . .*el aborto natural*
ehl ah-BOHR-toh nah-too-RAHL

ovary . . . .*el ovario*
ehl oh-VAH-ree-oh

placenta. . . . .*la placenta*
lah plah-SEHN-tah

pregnancy . . . .*el embarazo*
ehl ehm-bah-RAH-soh

reproductive . . . . *los órganos reproductivos*

CHILDBIRTH AND PREGNANCY—*continued*

organs   lohs OHR-gah-nohs
                             reh-proh-dooc-TEE-vohs

uterus . . . .*el útero*
                             ehl OO-teh-roh

First Steps in Pregnancy

Let's start by breaking the news of a pregnancy:

Congratulations! You are pregnant.
¡Felicidades! Está usted embarazada.
fch-lee-see-DAH-dehs. Ehs-TAH oos-
TEHD ehm-bah-rah-SAH-dah

You are ten weeks pregnant.
Está en la semana diez de embarazo.
ehs-TAH ehn lah seh-MAH-nah dee-EHS deh

If the patient does not look thrilled by the news, ask the following:

Would you like to consider other options?
¿Quiere considerar otras opciones?
kee-EH-reh cohn-see-deh-RAHR
OH-trahs op-see-OH-nehs

Some women may not welcome a pregnancy and ask for *un aborto* (oon ah-BOHR-toh), an abortion. Have some brochures in Spanish ready in your office that you can share with women facing this difficult decision.

Remember that you can always make a sentence negative by adding *no*: *No está usted embarazada* (You are not pregnant). The word *no* is also used in all the following negative commands.

Don't smoke while pregnant.
No fume cuando está embarazada.
noh FOO-meh KWAN-doh ehs-
TAH ehm-bah-rah-SAH-dah

Don't drink alcohol.
No beba alcohol.
noh BEH-bah ahl-coh-OHL

 Essential

To form the formal command of regular verbs, take the *–ar*, *–er*, or *–ir* ending of the verb and add the ending *–e* to *–ar* verbs and *–a* to *–er* and *–ir* verbs. For *fumar* (to smoke) you would say *fume* (smoke) or *no fume* (don't smoke). For *beber* (to drink), you would say *beba* (drink) or *no beba* (don't drink). Note that some verbs are irregular and do not follow this rule. An example is *salir* (to go out), *no salga* (don't go out).

Don't drink/consume too much caffeine.
No tome mucha cafeína.
no TOH-meh MOO-chah cah-feh-EE-nah

Don't take any medicines without consulting a doctor.
No tome medicinas sin consultar al doctor antes.
noh TOH-meh meh-dee-SEE-nahs seen cohn-sool-TAHR ahl doc-TOHR AHN-tehs

Here are some musts for *las mujeres embarazadas*, pregnant women.

Drink lots of water.
Beba mucho agua.
BEH-bah MOO-cha AH-goo-ah

Take prenatal vitamins
Tome vitaminas prenatales.
TOH-meh vee-tah-MEE-nahs preh-nah-TAH-lehs

Eat healthy food.
Coma comida saludable.
COH-mah coh-MEE-dah sah-loo-DAH-bleh

Healthy Pregnancies
Pregnant women visit the doctor regularly. To check their due date, ask the following:

When is your due date?
¿Cuándo es su día de parto?
KWAN-doh ehs soo DEE-ah deh PAHR-toh

Some women may have common pregnancy-related symptoms, such as *náusea* (nah-OO-seh-ah); *vómitos* (VOH-mee-tohs); *lloreras* (yoh-REH-rahs), frequent crying; and *fatiga* (fah-TEE-gah), fatigue. To check on other symptoms, say the following:

Do you have any vaginal discharge?
¿Tiene secreciones vaginales?
tee-EH-neh seh-creh-see-OH-nehs vah-hee-NAH-lehs

Call me or come if you have . . .
Llámeme o venga si tiene . . .
YAH-meh-meh oh VEHN-gah see tee-EH-neh . . .

PREGNANCY SYMPTOMS

constant	*vómitos continuos*
vomiting	VOH-mee-tohs cohn-tee-noo-OHS
blurred vision	*la vista nublada o borrosa*
	lah VEES-tah NOO-blah-dah oh
	boh-RROH-sah
dizziness	*mareos*
	mah-REH-ohs
fever	*fiebre*
	fee-EH-breh
swollen face	*la cara o dedos hinchados*
or fingers	lah CAH-rah oh DEH-dohs
	een-CHAH-dohs
spotting	*manchas de sangre*
	MAHN-chahs deh SAHN-greh

PREGNANCY SYMPTOMS—*continued*

painful	*dolor al orinar*
urination	doh-LOHR ahl oh-ree-NAHR
vaginal	*secreciones vaginales*
secretions	seh-creh-see-OH-nehs
	vah-hee-NAH-lehs
another	*otro síntoma que le preocupe*
symptom that	OH-troh SIN-toh-mah keh leh
worries you	pre-oh-COO-peh

Labor and Delivery

It's time! *Las contracciones*, contractions, have started and the patient has been admitted to the hospital. Start with these questions.

When did your contractions begin?
¿Cuándo comenzaron las contracciones?
KWAN-doh coh-mehn-SAH-rohn lahs
cohn-trac-see-OH-nehs

How many minutes apart are they now?
¿Cuántos minutos pasan entre contracciones ahora?
KWAN-tohs mee-NOO-tohs PAH-sahn EHN-treh
cohn-trac-see-OH-nehs ah-OH-rah

Has your water broken? When?
¿Se le ha roto la bolsa de aguas?¿Cuándo?
seh leh ah ROH-toh lah BOL-sah de
AH-goo-ahs. KWAN-doh

You can't drink or eat.
No puede beber o comer.
noh poo-EH-deh beh-BEHR oh coh-MEHR

If you are thirsty, eat ice chips.
Si tiene sed, coma pedacitos de hielo.
see tee-EH-neh sehd COH-mah peh-dah-SEE-tohs
deh ee-EH-loh

I have to examine you internally.
Tengo que hacerle un examen interno.
TEHN-goh keh ah-SEHR-leh oon EH-ksah-mehn
een-TEHR-noh

Put your legs in these stirrups.
Ponga los pies en estos estribos.
POHN-gah lohs pee-EHS ehn EHS-tohs
ehs-TREE-bohs

Spread your legs apart.
Abra las piernas.
AH-brah lahs pee-EHR-nahs

You are five centimeters dilated.
Está dilatada cinco centímetros.
ehs-TAH dee-lah-TAH-dah SEEN-coh
sehn-TEE-meh-trohs

Breathe.
Respire.
rehs-PEE-reh

Push!
¡Empuje!
ehm-POO-heh

Don't push now.
No empuje ahora.
noh ehm-POO-heh ah-OH-rah

For when the pain is getting too much to bear, you need to listen for your patient to say the following:

I want an epidural.
Quiero una epidural.
kee-EH-roh OO-nah eh-pee-doo-RAHL

Here are some phrases that will help you be ready in case there are *complicaciones* (com-plee-cah-see-OH-nehs), complications.

Your baby will be born prematurely.
Su bebé va a nacer prematuramente.
soo beh-BEH vah ah nah-SEHR
preh-mah-too-rah-MEHN-teh

This is a fetal monitor to hear the baby's heartbeat.
Esto es un monitor del feto para oír el latido del corazón del bebé.
EHS-toh ehs oon moh-nee-TOHR dehl FEH-toh PAH-rah oh-EER ehl lah-TEE-doh del coh-rah-SOHN dehl beh-BEH

We have to put an IV in your arm.
Le tenemos que poner un suero en el brazo.
leh teh-NEH-mohs keh poh-NEHR oon soo-EH-roh ehn ehl BRAH-soh

Your baby is in the breech position.
Su bebé está en una posición de nalgas.
soo beh-BEH ehs-TAH ehn OO-nah poh-see-see-OHN deh NAHL-gahs

You are not dilated enough.
No está dilatando lo suficiente.
noh ehs-TAH dee-lah-TAHN-doh loh soo-fee-see-EHN-teh

We are going to give you medicine so that you dilate faster.
Le vamos a dar medicina para que dilate más rápido.
leh VAH-mohs ah dahr meh-dee-SEE-nah PAH-rah keh dee-LAH-teh mahs RAH-pee-doh

We need to do a cesarean.
Tenemos que hacerle una cesárea.

teh-NEH-mohs keh AH-sehr-leh
OO-nah seh-SAH-reh-ah

If there are more serious complications, it is time to call *un/a intérprete* (oon/OO-nah een-TEHR-preh-teh), an interpreter.

There have been some more complications.
Ha habido más complicaciones.
ah ah-BEE-doh mahs com-plee-cah-see-OH-nehs

We will call an interpreter to explain it to you.
Vamos a llamar a un intérprete para que se lo explique.
VAH-mohs a yah-MAHR ah oon een-TEHR-preh-teh PAH-rah keh seh loh eks-PLEE-keh

But most of the time, you will hopefully be using:

Congratulations!
¡Felicidades!
feh-lee-see-DAH-dehs

You have a healthy baby!
¡Tiene un bebé sano!
tee-EH-neh oon beh-BEH SAH-noh

It's a boy!
¡Es un niño!
ehs oon NEE-nyoh

It's a girl!
¡Es una niña!
ehs OON-ah NEE-nyoh

 Alert!

Some people may not be familiar with pounds and ounces and may prefer to know the weight in kilos. One *libra* (LEE-brah), pound, is 454 *gramos* (GRAH-mohs), grams. One *kilo* (KEE-loh), kilo, is 2.2 *libras*, pounds. To convert pounds into kilos multiply the amount by 0.45. Seven pounds, for instance, would be 3.15 kilos.

Postpartum

New parents will probably be dying to know how heavy their new little family member is. *Pesar* (peh-SAHR) is "to weigh."

Your baby weighs seven pounds, ten ounces.
Su bebé pesa siete libras y diez onzas.
soo beh-BEH PEH-sah see-EH-teh LEE-brahs ee dee-EHS OHN-sahs

You should not have sex for six weeks.
No debe tener relaciones sexuales por seis semanas.
noh DEH-beh teh-NEHR reh-lah-see-OH-nehs se-ksoo-AH-lehs pohr seh-EEHS seh-MAH-nahs

If you have strong pains, call the doctor.
Si tiene dolores fuertes, llame al doctor.
see tee-EH-neh doh-LOH-rehs foo-EHR-tehs
YAH-meh ahl doc-TOHR

Do you want your baby circumcised?
¿Quiere que su bebé sea circuncidado?
kee-EH-reh keh soo beh-BEH SEH-ah
seer-coon-see-DAH-doh

Basic Baby and Child Care

Every culture has its own child-rearing practices. Before making any assumptions about child care, ask the following:

Do you have any questions about caring for your baby?
¿Tiene alguna pregunta sobre cómo cuidar al bebé?
tee-EH-neh ahl-GOO-nah preh-GOON-tah SOH-breh COH-moh coo-ee-DAHR ahl beh-BEH

Here is some basic baby care vocabulary:

BABY CARE

bottle . . . . *el biberón*
                    ehl bee-beh-ROHN
crib . . . . *la cuna*
                    la COO-nah

BABY CARE—*continued*

diaper	.*el pañal*
	ehl pah-NYAHL
drops	.*las gotas*
	lahs GOH-tahs
high chair	.*la silla alta*
	lah SEE-yah AHL-tah
lotion	.*la loción*
	lah loh-see-OHN
nipple	.*la tetina, el chupón*
(on a bottle)	lah teh-TEE-nah, ehl chooh-POHN
oil	.*el aceite*
	ehl ah-see-EE-teh
petroleum jelly	.*la jalea de petróleo*
	lah hah-LEH-ah deh peh-TROH-leh-oh
powder	.*el talco*
	ehl TAHL-coh

Feeding

Although breastfeeding is common in most Spanish-speaking countries, don't assume anything.

Are you planning to breastfeed your baby?
¿Piensa darle pecho a su bebé?
pee-EHN-sah DAHR-leh PE-choh ah soo beh-BEH

If your nipples bleed or crack, call your doctor.
Si le sangran o se le agrietan los pezones,
llame al doctor.

see leh SAHN-grahn oh seh leh ah-gree-EH-tahn
lohs peh-SOH-nehs, YAH-meh ahl doc-TOHR

According to the CDC National Immunization
Survey, 73.8 percent of babies born in the United
States in 2004 were breastfed at one time and
41.5 percent were still breastfeeding at six months
of age. To explain all the benefits of breastfeeding and to give instructions on how to breastfeed,
you can refer your patients to the Spanish version
of the *La Leche League* website: *www.llli.org/
langespanol.html*.

Your baby should eat every three hours.
Su bebé debe comer cada tres horas.
soo beh-BEH DEH-beh coh-MEHR
CAH-dah trehs OH-rahs

How many wet diapers did your baby have?
¿Cuántos pañales mojados tuvo su bebé?
KWAN-tohs pan-NYAH-lehs moh-HAH-
dohs TOO-voh soo beh-BEH

How many bowel movements did your baby have?
¿Cuántas evacuaciones tuvo su bebé?
KWAN-tahs eh-va-coo-ah-see-OH-nehs
TOO-voh soo beh-BEH

If you want to specify the period of time, you can add an adverb of time. Here are some options: *hoy* (OH-ee), today; *esta semana* (EHS-tah seh-MAH-nah), this week; *en los dos ultimos días* (ehn lohs dohs OOL-tee-mohs DEE-ahs), in the last two days.

Immunizations

In Spanish, vaccines are called *las vacunas* (lahs vah-COO-nahs), and the word for immunization is *la inmunización* (lah een-moo-nee-sah-see-OHN). To explain what immunization a child or adult needs, use the following:

> He/She needs a polio vaccine.
> *Necesita una vacuna contra el polio.*
> neh-seh-SEE-tah OO-nah vah-COO-nah
> COHN-trah ehl POH-lee-oh

ILLNESSES AND VACCINATIONS

Hepatitis A, B	.*la hepatitis A, B*
	lah eh-pah-TEE-tees ah, beh
DTaP (diphtheria,	.*la DTaP*
tetanus, acellular	la deh teh ah peh
pertussis)	
diphtheria	.*la difteria*
	lah deef-TEH-ree-ah
German measles. .	.*la rubeóla*
	lah roo-beh-OH-lah

ILLNESSES AND VACCINATIONS—*continued*

Hib (meningitis) . . . *HiB (la meningitis)*
                lah AH-cheh ee beh
                (lah meh-neen-HEE-tees)

influenza . . . . *la gripe*
                lah GREE-peh

IPB (polio) . . . . *la IPB (el polio)*
                lah ee peh beh (ehl POH-lee-oh)

MCV4 (bacterial . . . *MCV4 (la meningitis bacterial)*
meningitis)   lah meh-neen-HEE-tees
                bac-teh-ree-AHL

measles . . . . *el sarampión*
                chl sah-rahm-pee-OHN
                la EH-meh seh veh KWA-troh

mumps . . . . *la paroditis, las paperas*
                lah pah-roh-DEE-tees, lahs
                pah-PEH-rahs

PCV . . . . *la PCV*
(pneumococcal   lah peh seh veh
conjugate vaccine)

pertussis . . . . *la tos ferina*
                lah tohs feh-REE-nah

tetanus . . . . *el tétanos*
                ehl TEH-tah-nohs

varicella . . . . *la varicela*
(chicken pox)   lah vah-ree-SEH-lah

To explain what each vaccine is for, you can use *es para . . .* (It is to/for . . .).

It is to prevent bacterial infections.
Es para prevenir infecciones bacteriales.
ehs PAH-rah preh-veh-NEER een-fek-see-OH-nehs
bahc-teh-ree-AH-lehs

It is a vaccine to prevent German measles.
Es una vacuna para prevenir la rubeóla.
ehs OO-nah vah-COO-nah PAH-rah preh-veh-NEER
lah roo-beh-OH-lah

It needs to be given at two months old.
Hay que ponerla a los dos meses.
AH-ee keh poh-NEHR-lah ah lohs dohs MEH-sehs

This vaccine is recommended at two, four, and
six months.
*Se recomienda esta vacuna a los dos, cuatro y
seis meses.*
seh reh-coh-mee-EHN-dah EHS-tah vah-COO-nah
ah lohs dohs, KWAH-troh ee seh-EES MEH-sehs

Hepatitis B requires three injections.
La hepatitis B requiere tres inyecciones.
lah eh-pah-TEE-tees beh reh-kee-EH-reh trehs
een-yek-see-OH-nehs

Some patients may be worried about the safety of vaccines and may ask *¿Son seguras las vacunas?* (Are vaccines safe?).

It is uncommon for vaccines to cause a
serious reaction.
Es raro que las vacunas produzcan una reacción seria.
ehs RAH-roh keh lahs vah-COO-nahs proh-DOOS-
cahn OO-nah reh-ahk-see-OHN SEH-ree-ah

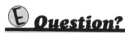

Question?

**What do I do when the patient requests more
information?**
Have some information available in Spanish. You can
print out brochures about immunizations at the CDC's
Spanish website, *www.cdc.gov/spanish/inmuniza-
cion.* If they do not request the information, you can
always offer it by saying *¿Quiere más información?*
(kee-EH-reh mahs cen-fohr-mah-see-OHN).

Some side effects are . . .
Algunos efectos secundarios son . . .
ahl-GOO-nohs eh-FEHK-tohs seh-coon-
DAH-ree-ohs sohn

SIDE EFFECTS

fever	*la fiebre*
	lah fee-EH-breh
redness	*la rojez*
	lah roh-HEHS
swelling	*la inflamación*
	lah een-flah-mah-see-OHN

Chapter 10
Emergency

If you work at the emergency room, you have probably seen it all. Now imagine having to react in Spanish. This chapter will arm you with some basic phrases and emergency vocabulary in Spanish.

How Did It Happen?

Whether you work at *la sala de emergencia* (lah SAH-lah deh eh-mehr-HEN-see-ah), the emergency room, or at a doctor's office, you will probably encounter different kinds of emergencies.

I am here to help you.
Estoy aquí para ayudarlo/la.
ehs-TOH-ee ah-KEE PAH-rah ah-yoo-DAHR-loh/lah

What happened?
¿Qué pasó?
keh pah-SOH

To find out the details, you can use the question words *dónde* (DOHN-deh), where; *cuándo* (KWAHN-doh), how; *cómo* (COH-moh), how; and *por qué* (pohr keh), why. Replace *qué* in *¿Qué pasó?* to modify the question.

EMERGENCIES

bee sting	*la picadura de abeja*
	lah pee-cah-DOO-rah deh ah-BEH-hah
dog bite	*la mordedura de perro*
	lah mohr-deh-DOO-rah deh PEH-rroh
fall	*la caída*
	lah cah-EE-dah
fire	*el incendio*
	ehl een-SEHN-dee-oh
frostbite	*el congelamiento*
	ehl cohn-heh-lah-mee-EHN-toh

EMERGENCIES—*continued*

gun shot . . . .*el disparo de arma de fuego*
ehl dees-PAH-roh deh AHR-mah deh
foo-EH-goh

heart attack . . . . . . *el ataque al corazón*
ehl ah-TAH-keh ahl coh-rah-SOHN

intoxication . . . . *la intoxicación*
lah een-toh-ksee-cah-see-OHN

overdose . . . . *la sobredósis*
lah soh-breh-DOH-sees

stabbing . . . . *la puñalada*
lah poo-NYAH-lah-dah

stroke . . . . *el derrame cerebral*
ehl deh-RRAH-meh seh-reh-BRAHL

suffocation . . . . *la sofocación*
lah soh-foh-cah-see-OHN

sun stroke . . . . *la insolación*
lah een-soh-lah-see-OHN

traffic accident . . . . *el accidente de tráfico*
ehl ak-see-DEHN-teh deh
TRAH-fee-coh

Admission Questions

Use the following basic admission questions when
you first see a patient:

Does anything hurt?
¿Le duele algo?
leh doo-EH-leh AHL-goh

Can you hear me? Nod your head.
¿Me puede oír? Asienta con la cabeza.
meh PWEH-deh oh-EER. ah-see-EHN-tah cohn lah
cah-BEH-sah

Is he/she conscious or unconscious?
¿Está consciente o inconsciente?
ehs-TAH cohn-see-EHN-teh oh een-cohn-see-EHN-teh

Please don't move.
Por favor no se mueva.
pohr fah-VOHR noh seh moo-EH-vah

Poisoning, Burns, and Broken Limbs

People come to the emergency room with conditions
varying from a *rasguños*, scrapes, to *hemorragia interna*,
internal hemorrhaging. Here is some basic vocabulary to
describe possible injuries:

INJURY TYPES

bruise. . . . .*el cardenal*
ehl cahr-deh-NAHL
burn . . . .*las quemadura*
lah keh-mah-DOO-rah
contusion. . . . .*la contusión*
lah cohn-too-see-OHN
cut . . . .*la cortada*
lah cohr-TAH-dah

INJURY TYPES—*continued*

dislocation. . . . .*la dislocación*
               lah dees-loh-cah-see-OHN

fracture . . . .*la fractura, la rotura*
               lah fract-TOO-rah, lah roh-TOO-rah

hemorrhage . . . . . .*la hemorragia*
               lah eh-moh-RRAH-hee-ah

scrape . . . .*el rasguño*
               ehl rahs-GOO-nyo

sprain. . . . .*la torcedura*
               lah tohr-seh-DOO-rah

wound . . . .*la herida*
               lah eh-REE-dah

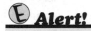 **Alert!**

In Spanish, there are several words to say "bruise," such as *el cardenal* (ehl cahr-deh-NAHL); *la moradura* (lah moh-rah-DOO-rah), used in Latin America; and *el moratón* (ehl moh-rah-TOHN), which is used in Spain. Another word used for *contusión* in this context is *el golpe* (ehl GOHL-peh).

Burns

A burn or a scald is called *la quemadura* (lah kehmah-DOO-rah). Use these phrases to deal with burn victims:

You have been burned.
Se ha quemado usted.
seh ah keh-MAH-doh oos-TEHD

What burned you?
¿Con qué se quemó?
cohn keh seh keh-MOH

BURN AGENTS

acid	*el ácido*
	ehl AH-see-doh
chemicals	*los productos químicos*
	lohs proh-DOOK-tohs KEE-mee-cohs
fire	*el fuego*
	ehl fee-EH-goh
gas	*el gas*
	ehl gahs
grease	*la grasa*
	lah GRAH-sah
hot water	*el agua caliente*
	ehl AH-goo-ah cah-lee-EHN-teh
oil	*el aceite*
	ehl ah-SEH-ee-teh
smoke	*el humo*
	ehl OOH-moh

Broken Limbs

In Spanish, a broken limb is described with the adjective as *roto/a* (ROH-toh/tah) or *fracturado/a* (frac-too-RAH-doh/dah), broken/fractured. Remember that in Spanish the gender of nouns and adjectives must agree, so it would be *el pie roto*, a broken foot, but *la muñeca rota*, a broken wrist.

You seem to have a broken arm.
Parece que tiene un brazo roto.
pah-REH-seh keh tee-EH-neh
oon BRAH-soh ROH-toh

You have a fractured leg.
Tiene una pierna fracturada.
tee-EH-neh OO-nah pee-EHR-nah frac-too-RAH-day

Other injury options are *dislocado/a* (dees-loh-CAH-doh/dah), dislocated; *distendido/a* (dees-tehn-DEE-doh/dah), pulled; and *torcido/a* (tohr-SEE-doh/dah), twisted.

You have a dislocated shoulder.
Tiene un hombro dislocado.
tee-EH-neh oon OHM-broh dees-loh-CAH-doh

You have a twisted ankle.
Tiene un tobillo torcido.
tee-EH-neh oon toh-BEE-yoh tohr-SEE-doh

You have a pulled muscle.
Tiene un músculo distendido.
tee-EH-neh oon MOOS-coo-loh dees-tehn-DEE-doh

Wounds

When there are *heridas* (eh-REE-dahs), wounds, use the following:

I am going to apply pressure to stop the bleeding.
Voy a aplicar presión para parar la sangre.
vohy ah ah-plee-CAHR preh-see-OHN
PAH-rah pah-RAHR lah SAHN-greh

You need stitches.
Necesita usted puntos.
neh-seh-SEE-tah oos-TEHD POON-tohs

Poisoning

Some signs of possible poisoning are *vómitos* (VOH-mee-tohs), vomiting; *olores inusuales* (oh-LOH-rehs ee-noo-soo-AH-lehs), unusual odors; *sudores* (soo-DOH-rehs), sweating; *manchas inusuales* (MAHN-chahs ee-noo-soo-AH-lehs), unusual stains; and *problemas al respirar* (proh-BLEH-mahs ahl rehs-pee-RAHR), trouble breathing.

What did you take?
¿Qué tomó?
keh toh-MOH

Did the substance get on your skin/eyes?
¿Hubo contacto de la sustancia con su piel/sus ojos?
OOH-boh cohn-TAC-toh deh lah soos-
TAHN-see-ah cohn soo pee-EHL

POISON AGENTS

alcohol	*el alcohol*
	ehl al-coh-OHL
ammonia	*el amoniaco*
	ehl ah-moo-nee-AH-coh
bleach	*el cloro*
	ehl CLOH-roh
cleaning product. .	*el producto de limpieza*
	ehl proh-DOOC-toh deh
	leem-pee-EH-sah
food	*la comida*
	lah coh-MEE-dah
insecticide.	*el insecticida*
	ehl een-sec-tee-SEH-day
lye.	*la lejía*
	lah leh-HEE-ah
mushrooms	*los hongos*
	lohs OHN-gohs
paint.	*la pintura*
	lah peen-TOO-rah
poison	*el veneno*
	ehl veh-NEH-noh
sleeping pills.	*los tranquilizantes*
	lohs trahn-kee-lee-SAHN-tehs

Overdose

If the patient is *consciente* (cons-see-EHN-teh), conscious, use the following phrases to assess the situation:

What drugs did you take?
¿Qué drogas tomó?
keh DOH-gahs toh-MOH

How much did you take?
¿Cuánto tomó?
KWAHN-toh toh-MOH

 Fact

According to the CDC, 95 percent of all unintentional poisoning deaths were caused by drugs. Pain medications were the most common cause, followed by cocaine and heroin

Were you trying to kill yourself?
¿Intentaba suicidarse?
een-tehn-TAH-bah soo-ee-see-DAHR-seh

DRUGS

amphetamines . . . .*las anfetaminas*
lahs ahn-feh-tah-MEE-nahs
barbiturates . . . . . .*los barbitúricos*
lohs bahr-bee-TOO-ree-cohs
cocaine . . . .*la cocaína, la coca*
lah coh-cah-EE-nah, lah COH-cah
crack . . . .*el crack*
ehl crahk

DRUGS—*continued*

crystal meth . . . . . . *el crystal meth, el cristal, la tina*
ehl CREES-tahl meth, ehl
creehs-TAHL, lah TEE-nah

ecstasy . . . . *el ecstasy*
ehl EHKS-tah-see

glue . . . . *el pegamento*
ehl peh-gah-MEHN-toh

hashish . . . . *el hachís*
ehl ah-CHEES

heroin . . . . *la heroína*
lah eh-roh-EE-nah

marijuana . . . . *la marihuana*
lah mah-ree-oo-AH-nah

morphine . . . . *la morfina*
lah mohr-FEE-nah

pain medications . . *los medicamentos para el dolor*
lohs meh-dee-cah-MEHN-tohs
PAH-rah ehl doh-LOHR

pills . . . . *las píldoras*
lahs PEEL-doh-rahs

speed . . . . *la metadrina*
lah meh-tah-DREE-nah

Heart Attack and Stroke

Los ataques al corazón (lohs ah-TAH-kehs ahl coh-rah-SOHN), heart attacks, and *los derrames cerebrales* (lohs deh-RRAH-mehs seh-reh-BRAH-lehs), strokes, are frequent causes of visits to the emergency room.

Do you have any of these symptoms?
¿Tiene alguno de estos síntomas?
tee-EH-nah ahl-GOO-noh deh EHS-
tohs SEEN-toh-mahs

Many of the symptoms below apply to heart attacks and strokes when they are *repentinos* (reh-pehn-TEE-nohs), sudden.

SYMPTOMS OF A HEART ATTACK

chest discomfort. . .*la molestia en el pecho*
lah moh-LEHS-tee-ah ehn
ehl PEH-choh

discomfort in. . . . . .*la molestia en la parte superior*
the upper body *del cuerpo*
lah moh-LEHS-tee-ah ehn lah
PAHR-teh soo-peh-ree-ohs dehl
coo-EHR-poh

dizziness . . . .*los mareos*
lohs mah-REH-ohs

nausea . . . .*las nauseas*
lahs NAH-oo-seh-ahs

shortness . . . .*la falta de aire*
of breath lah FAHL-tah deh ah-EE-reh

sweating . . . .*la sudoración*
la soo-doh-rah-see-OHN

SYMPTOMS OF A STROKE

loss of balance . . . . *la pérdida de equilibrio*
lah PEHR-dee-dah deh
eh-kee-LEE-bree-oh

numbness of the . . . *el entumecemiento del brazo,*
arm, face, or leg *la cara, o la pierna*
ehl ehn-too-meh-seh-mee-EHN-toh
dehl BRAH-soh, lah CAH-rah oh
lah pee-EHR-nah

severe headache . . . *el dolor de cabeza severo*
ehl doh-LOHR deh cah-BEH-sah
seh-VEH-roh

trouble seeing . . . . . *la dificultad para ver*
lah dee-fee-cool-TAHD PAH-rah vehr

trouble speaking . . *la dificultad para hablar*
lah dee-fee-cool-TAHD PAH-rah
ah-BLAHR

We are going to give you oxygen.
Le vamos a dar oxígeno.
leh VAH-mohs ah dahr oh-KSEE-heh-noh

We need to do a nuclear scan.
Tenemos que hacer un escáner nuclear.
teh-NEH-mohs keh ah-SEHR oon ehs-
CAH-nehr noo-cleh-AHR

We need to do a coronary angiography.
Tenemos que hacer una angiografía coronaria.

teh-NEH-mohs keh ah-SEHR OO-
nah ahn-hee-oh-grah-FEE-ah

Emergency Vocabulary

In case of emergency, you probably do not have time to get your phrase book out. Try to become familiar with these words beforehand:

EMERGENCY VOCABULARY

ambulance.......	*la ambulancia*
	lah ahm-boo-LAHN-see-ah
CPR.............	*la resucitación cardiopulmonar*
	lah reh-soo-see-tah-see-OHN
	cahr-dee-oh-pool-moh-NAHR
emergency.......	*el/la técnico de emergencia médica*
medical	ehl/lah TEHC-nee-coh deh eh-mehr-
technician	HEHN-see-ah MEH-dee-cah
first aid	*los primeros auxilios*
	lohs pree-MEH-rohs
	ah-oo-KSEE-lee-ohs
mouth-to-mouth ...	*la respiración boca a boca*
resuscitation	lah rehs-pee-rah-see-OHN BOH-cah
	ah BOH-cah
oxygen..........	*el oxígeno*
	ehl oh-KSEE-heh-noh
paramedic.......	*el/la paramédico/a*
	el/la pah-rah-MEH-dee-coh/cah
stitches	*los puntos* (Sp.), *las puntadas* (Lat. Am.)
	lohs POON-tohs, lahs poon-TAH-dahs

Here are some phrases you may want to use to inform the patient or relatives regarding what you are doing:

We need to do CPR.
Tenemos que hacer la resucitación cardiopulmonar.
teh-NEH-mohs keh ah-SEHR lah reh-soo-see-tah-see-OHN cahr-dee-oh-pool-moh-NAHR

We need stabilize the patient for transport.
Tenemos que estabilizar al/a la paciente.
teh-NEH-mohs keh ehs-tah-bee-lee-SAHR ahl/ah lah pah-see-EHN-teh

Essential

Recent immigrants may not be familiar with the basic emergency numbers in the United States. Share them. An example is, *En caso de emergencia, llame al 911* (ehn CAH-soh deh eh-mehr-HEHN-see-ah YAH-meh ahl noo-EH-veh OO-noh OO-noh), "In case of emergency call 911."

We need to get vital signs.
Tenemos que chequear los signos vitales.
teh-NEH-mohs keh cheh-keh-AHR
lohs SEEG-nohs vee-TAH-lehs

We need to apply a tourniquet.
Tenemos que hacer un torniquete.
teh-NEH-mohs keh ah-SEHR oon tohr-nee-KEH-teh

Chapter 11
Mental Health

You may have heard about *la vida loca*, the "crazy life," in a fun and harmless context. But the word *loco/a*, crazy, has intense negative connotations when in comes to dealing with mental health. Dealing with patients with mental health issues may be particularly challenging with Spanish-speaking patients who, because of cultural beliefs and values, may not acknowledge mental illness the same way you do.

Mental Health Professionals and Symptoms

First things first: introductions. There are different mental health care practitioners trained to treat mental illness. Remember that you can use *Soy . . .* (soy), meaning "I am," followed by the article and noun, to introduce yourself.

MENTAL HEALTH PRACTITIONERS

psychiatrist	*el/la psiquiatra*
	ehl/lah psee-kee-AH-trah
psychologist	*el/la psicólogo/a*
	ehl/lah psee-COH-loh-goh/gah
psychoanalyst	*el/la psicoanalista*
	ehl/lah psee-coh-ah-nah-LEES-tah
social worker	*el/la trabajador/a social*
	ehl/lah trah-bah-hah-DOHR/
	trah-bah-hah-DOH-rah soh-see-AHL
nurse practitioner	*el/la enfermero/a*
	ehl/lah ehn-fehr-MEH-roh/rah
pastoral counselor	*el/la consejero/a pastoral*
	ehl/lah cohn-seh-HEH-roh/
	rah pahs-toh-RAHL

Symptoms

Patients may come to you with a variety of symptoms. To check what symptoms they have ask the following:

What symptoms do you have?
¿Qué síntomas tiene?
keh SEEN-toh-mahs tee-EH-neh

Patients may reply with any of the following expressions using the verbs *sufrir* (suffer from) and *tener* (to have).

I suffer from panic attacks.
Sufro ataques de pánico.
SOO-froh ah-TAH-kehs deh PAH-nee-coh

I have anxiety.
Tengo ansiedad.
TEHN-goh ahn-see-eh-DAHD

Not all symptoms can be described with the verb *sufrir*, to suffer from. You would not say, for instance, *Sufro tristeza* (I suffer from sadness), but *Estoy triste* (I am sad).

SYMPTOMS

anxiety	*la ansiedad*
	lah ahn-see-eh-DAHD
catatonic behavior	*el comportamiento catatónico*
	ehl cohm-pohr-tah-mee-EHN-toh
	cah-tah-TOH-nee-coh
changes in appetite	*los cambios en el apetito*
	lohs CAHM-bee-ohs ehn ehl
	ah-peh-TEE-toh
delusions	*los delirios*
	lohs deh-LEE-ree-ohs
disorganized speech	*el lenguaje desorganizado*
	ehl lehn-goo-AH-heh dehs-ohr-
	gah-nee-SAH-doh

SYMPTOMS—*continued*

feelings of	*los sentimientos de impotencia*
helplessness	lohs sehn-tee-mee-EHN-tohs deh eem-poh-TEHN-see-ah
frequent loss	*la pérdida de estribos frecuente*
of temper	lah PEHR-dee-dah deh ehs-TREE-bohs freh-coo-EHN-teh
hallucinations	*las alucinaciones*
	lahs ah-oo-see-nah-see-OH-nehs
impaired	*el juicio afectado*
judgment	ehl hoo-EEH-see-oh ah-fec-TAH-doh
inability to sleep	*el no poder dormir*
	ehl noh poh-DEHR dohr-MEER
incoherence	*la incoherencia*
	lah een-coh-eh-REHN-see-ah
irritability	*la irritabilidad*
	lah ee-rree-tah-bee-lee-DAHD
lack of empathy	*la falta de empatía*
	lah FAHL-tah deh ehm-pah-TEE-ah
loss of energy	*la pérdida de energía*
	lah PEHR-dee-dah deh eh-nehr-HEE-ah
memory	*la deficiencia de memoria*
impairment	lah deh-fee-see-EHN-see-ah deh meh-moh-REE-ah
memory loss	*la pérdida de memoria*
	lah PEHR-dee-dah deh meh-MOH-ree-ah
mood swings	*los cambios de humor*
	lohs CAHM-bee-ohs deh ooh-MOHR

SYMPTOMS—*continued*

panic attacks......*los ataques de pánico*

lohs ah-TAH-kehs deh PAH-nee-coh

personality ....*los cambios de personalidad*
changes lohs CAHM-bee-ohs deh pehr-soh-

nah-lee-DAHD

sadness ....*la tristeza*

lah trees-TEH-sah

recurring ....*los pensamientos de muerte repetidos*
thoughts of death lohs pehn-sah-mee-EHN-tohs deh

moo-EHR-teh reh-peh-TEE-dohs

seizure...........*el ataque*

ehl ah-TAH-keh

violent behavior ...*el comportamiento violento*

ehl com-pohr-tah-mee-EHN-toh

vee-oh-LEHN-toh

 Essential

> *El no poder* literally translates as "the not being able
> to" and is used to describe symptoms of inability,
> such as *el no poder dormir* (inability to sleep) and *el
> no poder comer* (inability to eat). *La falta de*, which
> translates as "lack of," is used to describe symptoms
> where the patient lacks an ability, such as *la falta de
> autocontrol*, lack of self-control.

Here are some questions you can use to assess mental health status:

Why are you here?
¿Por qué está usted aquí?
pohr keh ehs-TAH oos-TEHD ah-KEE

Do you get messages from other places?
¿Recibe usted mensajes de otros lugares?
reh-SEE-bah oos-TEHD mehn-SAH-
hehs deh OH-trohs loo-GAH-rehs

Do you hear any voices?
¿Oye usted voces?
Oh-yeh oos-TEHD VOH-sehs

Do you forget things?
¿Se le olvidan cosas?
seh leh ol-VEE-dahn COH-sahs

Have you ever thought about wanting to die?
¿Alguna vez ha pensado en querer morir?
ahl-GOO-nah vehs ah pehn-SAH-
doh ehn keh-REHR MOH-reer

Have you ever thought that life is too hard?
*¿Alguna vez ha pensado que la vida es
demasiado dura?*
ahl-GOO-nah vehs ah pehn-SAH-doh keh lah
VEE-dah ehs deh-mah-see-AH-doh DOO-rah

How is your memory?
¿Qué tal está su memoria?
keh tahl ehs-TAH soo meh-MOH-ree-ah

How is your sexual interest or desire?
¿Cómo está su interés o deseo sexual?
COH-moh ehs-TAH soo een-teh-REHS
oh deh-SEH-oh seh-ksoo-AHL

Some of the possible answers to the last two questions are *bien* (bee-EHN), well, *normal* (nohr-MAHL), normal, or *no tengo interés* (noh TEHN-goh een-teh-REHS), I don't have any interest. To check the patient's mood state use the following:

What is your mood most of the time?
¿Cómo está de estado de ánimo la
mayor parte del tiempo?
COH-moh ehs-TAH deh ehs-TAH-doh deh AH-nee-moh lah mah-YOHR PAHR-teh dehl tee-EHM-poh

POSSIBLE MOOD STATES

euphoric . . . . *eufórico*
eh-oo-FOH-ree-coh
depressive . . . . *depresivo*
deh-preh-SEE-voh
irritable . . . . *irritable*
ee-rree-TAH-bleh
low . . . . *bajo*
BAH-hoh

POSSIBLE MOOD STATES—*continued*

normal . . . .*normal*

nohr-MAHL

On some occasions you will have to deal with relatives rather than the patients themselves.

How has the patient's behavior changed?
¿Cómo ha cambiado el comportamiento del/
de la paciente?
COH-moh ah cahm-bee-AH-doh ehl com-pohr-tah-mee-EHN-toh dehl/deh lah pah-see-EHN-teh

Has anyone in the family had mental illness?
¿Ha tenido alguien de la familia enfermedad mental?
ah teh-NEE-doh ahl-ghee-EHN deh lah fah-MEE-lee-ah ehn-fehr-meh-DAHD MEHN-tahl

Mental health assessment and treatment may be affected by factors other than language. Asking about any other advice the family has sought may help you assess their beliefs and approaches.

Who have you consulted with?
¿Con quién ha consultado usted?
cohn kee-EHN ah cohn-sool-TAH-doh oos-TEHD

Some of the answers may include an *espiritista*, *santero/a*, or *curandero/a*, a folk healer. Other families may also be influenced by their religion and may want to include *el cura* (ehl COO-rah), priest, in the process. It is important to assess and respect the values or beliefs of the patient before suggesting your approach.

What did he/she say?
¿Qué le dijo?
keh leh DEE-hoh

 Essential

Mental status exams often include questions that are culturally biased. Some tests assess the patient's general fund of knowledge to get a sense of his or her ability to store information or sense of reality. It would, however, be unfair to ask a recent immigrant to name American presidents or U.S. state capitals. Take the patient's background and language ability into account.

Conditions

To share the news of a diagnosis, you can use the following phrases.

You have depression.
Tiene usted depresión.
tee-EH-neh oos-TEHD deh-preh-see-OHN

We think it is autism.
Creemos que es autismo.
creh-EH-mohs keh ehs ah-oo-TEES-moh

Here is a list of possible conditions:

CONDITIONS

ADHD, attention deficit hyperactivity disorder	*TDAH, el transtorno por déficit de atención con hiperactividad* teh, deh, ah, AH-cheh; ehl trahns-TOHR-noh pohr DEH-fee-seet deh ah-ten-see-OHN cohn ee-pehr-ac-tee-vee-DAHD
Alzheimer's disease	*la enfermedad de Alzheimer* lah ehn-fehr-med-DAHD deh ahl-tzah-EE-mehr
anxiety disorder	*el transtorno de ansiedad generalizada* ehl trans-TOHR-noh deh an-see-EH-dahd heh-neh-rah-lee-SAH-dah
autism	*el autismo* ehl ah-oo-TEES-moh
bipolar disorder	*la enfermedad bipolar* lah ehn-fehr-meh-DAHD bee-poh-LAHR
dementia	*la demencia* lah deh-MEHN-see-ah
depression	*la depresión* lah deh-preh-see-OHN
epilepsy	*la epilepsia* lah eh-pee-LEP-see-ah
obsessive compulsive behavior	*el transtorno de comportamiento obsesivo compulsivo* ehl trans-TOHR-noh deh com-pohr-tah-mee-EHN-toh ob-seh-SEE-voh

CONDITIONS—*continued*

personality	*el transtorno de personalidad*
disorder	ehl trans-TOHR-noh deh deh
	pehr-soh-nah-lee-DAHD
PTSD, post-.	*el transtorno de estrés postraumático*
traumatic stress	ehl trahns-tohr-noh deh ehs-TREHS
disorder	pohs-trah-oo-MAH-tee-coh
schizophrenia	*la esquizofrenia*
	lah ehs-kee-soh-FREH-nee-ah

 Alert!

When talking about mental health, disease can be translated as *la enfermedad* (lah ehn-fehr-meh-DAHD) or *el transtorno* (ehl trans-TOHR-noh). *Transtorno* can also translate as "disorder". Alzheimer's disease, for instance, can be *la enfermedad de Alzheimer* or *el transtorno de Alzheimer*.

Eating Disorders

Many people suffer from *los transtornos de la alimentación* (lohs trans-TOHR-nohs deh ah-lee-mehn-tah-see-OHN), eating disorders.

EATING DISORDERS

anorexia	*la anorexia*
	lah ah-noh-REHK-see-ah
bulimia.	*la bulimia*
	lah boo-LEEH-mee-ah

EATING DISORDERS—*continued*

compulsive	*el comer compulsivamente*
eating	ehl coh-MEHR com-pool-SEE-vah-mehn-teh

EATING DISORDER SYMPTOMS

excessive	*la preocupación excesiva por el peso*
worrying	lah preh-oh-coo-pah-see-OHN
about weight	ex-seh-SEE-vah pohr ehl PEH-soh
excessive	*el hacer demasiado ejercicio*
exercising	ehl ah-SEHR deh-mah-see-AH-doh eh-hehr-SEE-see-oh
obsessing about . .	*la obsesión con las calorías*
calories	lah ob-seh-see-OHN cohn lahs cah-loh-REE-ahs
use of medicines . .	*el uso de medicamentos para*
to prevent	*prevenir el aumento de peso*
weight gain	ehl OO-soh deh meh-dee-cah-MEHN-tohs PAH-rah preh-veh-NEER ehl ah-oo-MEHN-toh deh PEH-soh
voluntary	*el vomitar voluntario*
vomiting	ehl voh-mee-TAHR ex-seh-SEE-voh

Treatment Options

There are usually several options when it comes to treatment of mental health conditions. It is important that the patient understands that there may be a choice.

You have different options.
Tiene usted varias opciones.
tee-EH-neh oos-TEHD VAH-ree-ahs op-see-OH-nehs

Therapy Types

In Spanish, therapy is *la terapia* (lah teh-RAH-pee-ah). Patients may choose to go to *la terapia de parejas* (lah teh-RAH-pee-ah deh pah-REH-hahs), couple's therapy, *la terapia de familia* (lah teh-RAH-pee-ah deh fah-MEE-lee-ah), or *la terapia individual* (lah teh-RAH-pee-ah een-dee-vee-doo-AHL).

THERAPIES

behavior therapy	*la terapia de comportamiento* lah teh-RAH-pee-ah deh com-pohr-tah-mee-EHN-toh
drug therapy	*la terapia con medicamentos* lah teh-RAH-pee-ah cohn meh-dee-cah-MEHN-tohs
electroconvulsive therapy	*la terapia electroconvulsiva* lah teh-RAH-pee-ah eh-lehc-troh-cohn-vool-SEE-vah
hypnotherapy	*la hipnoterapia* lah eep-noh-teh-RAH-pee-ah
psychotherapy	*la psicoterapia* lah psee-coh-teh-RAH-pee-ah

Here are some of the most common medication types prescribed for mental health conditions:

MEDICATIONS

anti-anxiety . . . . . .*las drogas contra la ansiedad*
drugs   lahs DROH-gahs COHN-trah lah
             ahn-see-eh-DAHD

anticonvulsant . . . .*el anticonvulsivante*
             ehl ahn-tee-cohn-vool-see-VAHN-teh

antidepressant . . . .*el antidepresivo*
             ehl ahn-tee-deh-preh-SEE-voh

antipsychotic. . . . . .*el antipsicótico*
             ehl ahn-tee-psee-COH-tee-coh

 Question?

What do I say if I need help?
If you need the relatives or some colleagues to help you with a patient, you can always say *¿Puede ayudarme, por favor?* (PWEH-deh ah-yoo-DAHR-meh pohr fah-VOHR), "Can you help me, please?" If the situation is more urgent, a loud *¡Ayuda!* (ah-YOO-dah), "Help!" may do it.

Hospitalization and Commitment

In some cases, the patient may have to *ser hospitalizado/a* (sehr ohs-pee-tah-lee-SAH-doh/dah), be hospitalized. These phrases will help you convey the idea.

You are restricted to this area.
No puede usted salir de esta área.
noh poo-EH-deh sah-LEER deh EHS-tah AH-reh-ah

You are on a thirty-six-hour hold.
Usted tiene que quedarse aquí treinta y seis horas.
oos-TEHD tee-EH-neh keh keh-DAHR-seh
ah-KEE treh-EEN-tah ee seys OH-rahs

Routine medications are given at 8 A.M., 2 P.M.,
and 6 P.M.
*Se dan medicinas de rutina a las ocho, a las
dos y a las seis.*
seh dahn meh-dee-SEE-nahs deh roo-TEE-nah
ah lahs OH-choh, ah lahs dohs ee ah lahs seys

Appendix A

English-Spanish Dictionary

abdomen
el abdomen

abortion
el aborto

address
la dirección

ADHD
TDAH, el transtorno por déficit de atención con hiperactividad

adhesive tape/plaster
la cinta adhesiva/el espadadrapo

bandage
la venda

age
la edad

AIDS
el SIDA

alcohol
el alcohol

all the time
todo el tiempo

allergic reactions
las reacciones alérgicas

alternative treatments
los tratamientos alternativos

Alzheimer's disease
la enfermedad de Ahlzeimer

American
estadounidense

analgesic
el analgésico

anemia
la anemia

anesthesia
la anestesia

anesthesiologist
el/la anestesiólogo/a

anesthesiology
la anestesiología

angiogram
el angiograma

animal allergy
la alergia a los animales

ankle
el tobillo

anorexia
la anorexia

antacid
el antiácido

anti-inflammatory
el antiinflamatorio

anti-anxiety drugs
las drogas contra la ansiedad

antiarrhythmic
la medicina antiarrítmica

antibiotic
el antibiótico

antibiotics allergy
la alergia a los antibióticos

anticoagulant
el anticoagulante

anticonvulsant
el anticonvulsivante

antidepressant
el antidepresivo

antidiarrheal
el antidiarréico

anti-emetics
el antiemético

antifungal
el antifúngico

antihypertensive
el antihipertensivo

antineoplastic
el antineoplásico

antipsychotic
el antipsicótico

antipyretic
el antipirético

antiviral
la medicina antiviral

anxiety
la ansiedad

anxiety disorder
el transtorno de ansiedad generalizada

appointment
la cita

April
abril

Argentinean
argentino/a

arm
el brazo

armpit
la axila, el sobaco

arteriography
la arteriografía

arthritis
el artritis

aspirin
la aspirina

asthma
el asma

August
agosto

aunt
la tía

autism
el autismo

available
disponible

back
la espalda

backache
dolor de espalda

bacterial
bacterial

barbiturate
el barbitúrico

bassinet
el moisés

bathroom
los servicios (Sp.), el baño

be
ser, estar

bed
la cama

bedpan
el orinal

behavior therapy
la terapia de comportamiento

bevavior
el comportamiento

bipolar disorder
la enfermedad bipolar

birth control patch
el parche anticonceptivo

blister
la ampolla

blood pressure
la tensión sanguínea

blood transfusion
la transfusión de sangre

blood type
el grupo sanguíneo

body fat percentage
el porcentaje de grasa del cuerpo

Bolivian
boliviano/a

bottle
el biberón

boyfriend/girlfriend
el/la novio/a

break water
romper la bolsa de agua

breast cancer
el cáncer de pecho/seno

breast
el pecho, el seno

breastfeed
dar el pecho, dar el seno, amamantar

breath
respirar

brochure
el folleto

bronchitis
la bronquitis

bronchoscopy
la broncoscopia

brother/sister
el/la hermano/a

brother/sister-in-law
el/la cuñado/a

bulimia
la bulimia

burning sensation
el ardor

buttocks
la nalga

cafeteria
la cafetería

call
llamar

call bell
el timbre

cancer
el cáncer

carbohydrates
los carbohidratos

cardiac catheterization
la cateterización cardíaca

cardiograph
el cardiógrafo

cardiologist
el/la cardiólogo/a

cardiology
la cardiología

cashier
el cajero

catatonic behavior
el comportamiento catatónico

catheter
el catéter, la sonda

cervical cancer
el cáncer cervical/cérvico

cervical cap
el capuchón cervical

cervical dysplasia
la displasia cervical

cesarean section
la operación cesárea

change in lifestyle
el cambio en el estilo de vida

changes in appetite
los cambios en el apetito

chapel
la capilla

cheek
la mejilla

chemotherapy
la quimoterapia

chest
el pecho

chewtab
la tableta masticable

Chilean
chileno/a

chills
los escalofríos

chin
el mentón (Lat. Am.), la barbilla (Sp.)

Chlamydia
la clamidia

cholecystectomy
la colecistectomía

circulatory system
el sistema circulatorio

city
la ciudad

clean
limpiar, limpio/a

cleanser
el limpiador

codeine
la codeína

cold remedy
el remedio contra el resfriado

Colombian
colombiano/a

complication
la complicación

compulsive eating
el comer compulsivamente

computed tomography or CT scan
la tomografía computerizada

condom
el condón, el preservativo masculino

conscious or intravenous sedation
la sedación consciente or intravenosa

consent
el consentimiento

constant
constante

container
el container, el frasco/frasquito

contraction
la contracción

cosmetic surgery
la cirugía cosmética

Costa Rican
costarricense

cotton swabs
los palitos de algodón

cough
toser

cough suppressant
el supresor de tos

counselor
el/la consejero/a

cousin
el/la primo/a

cover
cubrir

coworker
el/la colega

crib
la cuna

crutches
las muletas

Cuban
cubano/a

curative surgery
la cirugía curativa

curette
la cureta

daily
todos los días

date
la fecha

date of birth
la fecha de nacimiento

daughter
hija

daughter-in-law
la nuera

day
el día

December
diciembre

decision
la decisión

decongestant
el descongestionante

delivery
el parto

delusions
los delirios

dementia
la demencia

Depo-Provera injection
la inyección Depo Provera

depression
la depresión

depressive
depresivo

dermatologist
el/la dermatólogo/a

dermatology
la dermatología

diabetes
el/la diabetes

diagnostic surgery
la cirugía diagnóstica

diaper
el pañal

diaphragm
el diafragma

die, pass away
fallecer

digestive system
el sistema digestivo

diphtheria
la difteria

discharge
dar de alta

disorganized speech
el lenguaje desorganizado

dizzy
mareado/a

Dominican
dominicano/a

donate
donar

dose
la dósis

dripping
el goteo

drops
las gotas

drug therapy
la terapia con medica-mentos

drugs
las drogas

DTaP (diphtheria, tetanus, acellular pertussis)
la DTaP

dust allergy
la alergia al polvo

ear
la oreja (external)/el oído (internal)

earache
dolor de oído

ECG monitor
el monitor del electrocardiograma

ECP emergency contraceptive pills
la píldora del día después

Ecuadorian
ecuatoriano/a

EEG
el electroencefalograma

effeverescent table
la tableta efervescente

eighth
octavo

EKG or ECG
el electrocardiograma

El Salvadoran
salvadoreño/a

elbow
el codo

elective surgery
la cirugía opcional

electrocardiograph
el electrocardiógrafo

electroconvulsive therapy
la terapia electroconvulsiva

elevator
el elevador (Lat. Am.), el ascensor (Sp.)

e-mail
email; el mail, el correo electrónico

emergency contact
el contacto de emergencia

emergency exit
la salida de emergencia

emergency kit
el botiquín de emergencia

emergency room
la sala de emergencia

emergency surgery
la cirugía de emergencia

endocrine system
el sistema endocrino

endocrinologist
el/la endicronólogo/a

endocrinology
la endicronología

endoscopy
la endoscopia

endurance
la resistencia física

enema
el enema

English
el inglés

epidural
la anestesia epidural

epilepsy
la epilepsia

episiotomy
la episotomía

euphoric
eufórico

examine
examinar

excessive bleeding
el sangrar excesivamente

exit
la salida

experimental treatment
el tratamiento experimental

eye
el ojo

face
la cara

faint
desmayarse

fallopian tubes
las trompas de falopio

family
la familia

fat
las grasas, gordo/a, obeso/a

father/mother
el padre/la madre

father/mother-in-law
el/la suegro/a

February
febrero

feelings of helplessness
los sentimientos de impotencia

female condom
el condón femenino

female sterilization
la esterilización femenina

fertility awareness
el método del ritmo

fiancé/fiancée
el/la prometido/a

fifth
quinto

Filipino/a
filipino/a

finger
el dedo

first
primer

flexibility
la flexibilidad

floor
el piso

foam
la espuma

food poisoning
la intoxicación alimentaria

foot
el pie

forearm
el antebrazo

forehead
la frente

fourth
cuarto

frequent loss of temper
la pérdida de estribos frecuente

Friday
viernes

friend
el/la amigo/a

fungal
de hongos

gag
tener arcadas

gastroenteritis
la gastrointeritis

gastrointestinal system
*el sistema gastrointes-
tinal*

gel
la crema, el gel

gel capsule
la cápsula de gel

German measles
la rubeóla

glaucoma
el glaucoma

gonorrhea
la gonorrea

gout
la gota

grandfather/grand-
mother
el/la abuelo/a

grandson/granddaugh-
ter
el/la nieto/a

Guatemalan
guatemalteco/a

gynecologist
el/la ginecólogo/a

gynecology
la ginecología

hallucinations
las alucinaciones

hand
la mano

have
tener

have a bowel movement
evacuar

head
la cabeza

healthy
sano/a, saludable

heart disease
*las enfermedades del
corazón*

heel
el talón

height
la altura

hepatitis A, B, C
la hepatitis A, B, C

hernia
la hernia

herpes
el herpes

hi
hola

Hib (meningitis)
HiB (la meningitis)

high chair
la silla alta

high/low blood pressure
*la presión sanguínea
alta/baja*

high/low cholesterol
el colesterol alto/bajo

hip
la cadera

HIV
el HIV

hives
la urticaria

Honduran
hondureño/a

hormone
la hormona

hot flashes
*la sensación de calor
intenso*

hour
la hora

HPV
*una infección genital
por VPH*

hurt
doler

husband/wife
el/la esposo/a

hypertension
la hipertensión

hypnotherapy
la hipnoterapia

hypodermic needle
la hipodérmica

hypoglycemia
la hipoglucemia

hysterectomy
la histerectomía

ibuprofen
el ibuprofeno

ice pack
la bolsa de hielo

immunosuppressant
el inmunosupresor

impaired judgment
el juicio afectado

improve
mejorar

inability to sleep
el no poder dormir

incoherence
la incoherencia

indigestion
la indigestión

infection
la infección

inflatable cuff
la abrazadera hinchable

influenza, flu
la gripe

inhaler
el inhalador

injection
la inyección

insect sting allergy
la alergia a las picaduras de insectos

insurance
el seguro médico

insurance company
la compañía de seguros

intensive care
los cuidados intensivos

interpreter
el/la intérprete

IPB (polio)
la IPB (el polio)

irritability
la irritabilidad

irritable
irritable

irritation
la irritación

itch
picar

itchiness
el picor

IUD
el DIU (el dispositivo intrauterino)

January
enero

jaw
la mandíbula

July
julio

June
junio

kidney stones
las piedras en el riñón

knee
la rodilla

labor pains
los dolores del parto

laboratory
el laboratorio

lack of empathy
la falta de empatía

laparoscopic surgery
la laparoscopia

laryngitis
la laringitis

laser surgery
la operación de láser

laxative
el laxativo, el laxante

leg
la pierna

leukemia
la leucemia

lip
el labio

local anesthesia
la anestesia local

look for
buscar

loss of energy
la pérdida de energía

lotion
la loción

low
bajo

lump
el bulto

lupus
el lupus

main lobby
la sala principal

major surgery
la cirugía mayor

mammogram
el mamograma

March
marzo

marital status
el estado civil

mastectomy
la mastectomía

maternity ward
la sala de maternidad

May
mayo

measles
el sarampión

measure
medir

medical form
el formulario médico

medical student
el/la estudiante de medicina

medication
la medicación

medicine
la medicina

memory impairment
la deficiencia de memoria

memory loss
la pérdida de memoria

meningitis
la meningitis

menopause
la menopausia

menstruation
el periodo, la menstruación

Mexican
mexicano/a

microscope
el microscopio

microsurgery
la microcirugía

midwife
el comadrón/la comadrona

migraine
la migraña

minerals
los minerales

minor
menor de edad

minor surgery
la cirugía menor

minute
el minuto

miscarriage
el aborto natural

moderately
moderadamente

Monday
lunes

monitor
el monitor

month
el mes

mood swings
los cambios de humor/genio

morphine
la morfina

mouth
la boca

MRI
la imagen por resonancia magnética

mucus
la mucosidad

mumps
la parotiditis, las paperas

muscle relaxant
el relajante de músculos

muscular strength
la fortaleza muscular

nail
la uña

name
el nombre

nasal spray
el aerosol, el spray

natural remedies
los remedios naturales

neck
el cuello

need
necesitar

negative
negativo

neighbor
el/la vecino/a

nephew/niece
el/la sobrino/a

nervous system
el sistema nervioso

neurologist
el/la neurólogo/a

neurology
la neurología

never
nunca

Nicaraguan
nicarangüense

night sweats
los sudores nocturnos

ninth
noveno

nipple
el pezón

nipple (on a bottle)
la tetina, el chupón

normal
normal

nose
la nariz

November
noviembre

number
el número

numbness
el entumecimiento

nurse/nurse practitioner
el/la enfermero/a

nurse's aid
*el/la asistente de
enfermero*

nutrition
la nutrición

nutritionist
el/la nutricionista

observe
observar

obsessive compulsive
behavior
*el transtorno de com-
portamiento obsesivo
compulsivo*

obstetrician
el/la obstetra

obstetrics
obstetricia

occasionally
de vez en cuando

occupation
la profesión

October
octubre

oil
el aceite

ointment
el ungüento

oncologist
el/la oncólogo/a

oncology
la oncología

operate
operar

ophthalmologist
el/la oftalmólogo/a

ophthalmology
la oftalmología

ophthalmoscope
el oftalmoscopio

organ donor
el/la donante de órganos

orthopedist
el/la ortopedista

orthopedics
la ortopedia

osteoporosis
la osteoporosis

otorhinolaryngologist
el/la otorrinolaringólogo/a

ounce
la onza

ovarian cancer
*(el) cáncer de ovario/
ovárico*

ovarian cysts
quistes en el ovario

ovary
el ovario

over-sedation
la sedación excesiva

oxygen supply device
*el aparato para el sumin-
istro de oxígeno*

pail (for diapers)
el balde para pañales

painful
doloroso/a

palliative surgery
la cirugía paliativa

Panamanian
panameño/a

panic attacks
los ataques de pánico

Paraguayan
payaguayo/a

parking lot
el estacionamiento

Parkinson's disease
*la enfermedad de Parkin-
son, el Parkinson's*

pastoral counselor
el/la consejero/a pastoral

patch
el parche

patient
el/la paciente

patient's chart
la ficha del paciente

PCV (pneumococcal
conjugate vaccine)
la PCV

peanut allergy
*la alergia a los caca-
huetes*

pediatrician
el/la pediatra

pelvic exam
el exámen pélvico

pelvic inflammatory
disease
*(la) enfermedad inflama-
toria pélvica*

penis
el pene

permission
el permiso

personality changes
*los cambios de person-
alidad*

personality disorder
*el transtorno de person-
alidad*

pertussis
la tos ferina

Peruvian
peruano/a

petroleum jelly
la jalea de petróleo

pharmacist
el/la farmacéutico/a

phlegm
la flema

phone number
el número de teléfono

physical therapist
el/la terapeuta físico/a

physical therapy
la terapia física

physician's assistant
el/la asistente de médico

pill
la píldora, la pastilla

pipette
la pipera

place of employment
el lugar de empleo

placenta
la placenta

plastic surgery
la cirugía plástica

pneumonia
la neumonía

policy holder
el/la titular de la póliza

polio
el polio

pollen allergy
la alergia al polen

positive
positivo

pound
la libra

powder
el talco

pregnancy
el embarazo

pressure
presionar

preventive surgery
la cirugía preventiva

protect
proteger

protein
las proteínas

psychiatrist
el/la psiquiatra

psychiatry
la psiquiatría

psychoanalyst
el/la psicoanalista

psychologist
el/la psicólogo/a

psychotherapy
la psicoterapia

PTSD, post-traumatic
stress disorder
*el transtorno de estrés
postraumático*

Puerto Rican
puertorriqueño/a

punctured organs
*las perforaciones en los
órganos*

radiation shield
el escudo antirradiación

radiation theraphy
la terapia de radiación

radiologist
el/la radiólogo/a

radiology
la radiología

rarely
rara vez

rash
el salpullido

reaction
la reacción

reception area
*el área de recepción, la
recepción*

receptionist
el/la recepcionista

recovery room
la sala de recuperación

recurring thoughts of death
los pensamientos de muerte repetidos

reflex hammer
el martillo de reflejos

regional anesthesia
la anestesia regional/ parcial

relative
el/la familiar/el/la pariente/a

relieve
aliviar

remove
extirpar

reproductive organs
los órganos reproductivos

reproductive system
el sistema reproductivo

required surgery
la cirugía requerida

resources
los recursos

respiratory system
el sistema respiratorio

resting heart rate
el pulso en descanso

restore
reposicionar

result
el resultado

ring
el anillo vaginal

ringworm
la tiña

risk
el riesgo

robe
la bata

robotic surgery
la cirugía robótica

sadness
la tristeza

saliva
la saliva

sample
la muestra

sangrar
to bleed

Saturday
sábado

scale
la escala, el peso

scarlet fever
la escarlatina

schizophrenia
la esquizofrenia

second
segundo

secretary
el/la secretario/a

sedative
el sedativo

see
ver

seizure
el ataque

September
septiembre

seventh
séptimo

shellfish allergy
la alergia al marisco

shin
la espinilla

sinusitis
la sinusitis

sixth
sexto

skin
la piel

sleeping drug
la droga para dormir

smell
oler

smell
el olor

smoke
fumar

social security number
el número de la seguro social

social worker
el/la trabajador/a social

sole
la planta del pie

sometimes
a veces

son/daughter
el/la hijo/a

son-in law
el yerno

sores
las llagas

soy allergy
la alergia a la soja

Spanish
el español

Spanish
español/española

speak
hablar

specialist
el/la especialista

speech therapist
el/la terapeuta de lenguaje

sphygmomanometer
el baumanómetro

spirometer
el espirómetro

spit
escupir

sputum
el esputo

staple
la grapa

state
el estado

stepbrother/stepsister
el/la hermanastro/a

stepfather/stepmother
el padrastro/la madrastra

stepson/stepsister
el/la hijastro/a

sterilized gauze
la gasa esterilizada

stethoscope
el estetoscopio

stitches
los puntos, las puntadas

stomach
el estómago

stool
el excremento

stress
el estrés

stretcher
la camilla

stroke
el derrame cerebral

Sunday
domingo

suppository
el supositorio

surgeon
el/la cirujano/a

surgery
la operación, la cirugía

swallow
tragar

sweat
sudar

swollen
hinchado/a

syphilis
(la) sífilis

syringe
la jeringa, la jeringuilla

syrup
el jarabe

tablet
la pastilla

tachycardia
la taquicardia

telephone
el teléfono

tenth
décimo

testicle
el testículo

tetanus
el tétanos

therapist
el/la terapeuta

thermometer
el termómetro

thigh
el muslo

third
tercer

throat
la garganta

thumb
el pulgar

Thursday
jueves

thyroid disease
la enfermedad de tiroides

timer
el microcronómetro

to apply
aplicar

to attach
pegar

to chew
masticar

to deliver
dar a luz, parir

to insert
meter

to put
poner

to spray
rociar

to take
tomar

toe
el dedo del pie

tongue
la lengua

tongue depressor
el bajalengua

tooth
el diente

toothache
dolor de muelas

touch
tocar

tourniquet
el torniquete

tranquilizer
el tranquilizante

transplant
transplantar, el transplante

treatment
el tratamiento

tubal litigation
la ligadura tubárica

tuberculosis, TB
la tuberculosis

Tuesday
martes

ulcer
la úlcera

ultrasound
la ecografía, el ultrasound

uncle
el tío

urinary incontinence
la incontinencia

urinary track infection
cistitis

urinate
orinar

urologist
el/la urólogo/a

urology
la urología

Uruguayan
uruguayo/a

uterine fibroids
el fibroma uterino

uterus
el útero

vagina
la vagina

vaginal discharge
las secreciones vaginales

vaginal spermicides
los espermicidas vaginales

varicella (chicken pox)
la varicela

vasectomy
la vasectomía

Venezuelan
venezolano

violent behavior
el comportamiento violento

viral
vírica

vital signs
los signos vitales

vitamin
la vitamina

waist
la cintura

wait
esperar

waiting room
la sala de espera

warts
las verrugas

wash
lavar

water fountain
la fuente

Wednesday
miércoles

week
la semana

weigh
pesar

weight
el peso

weight gain/loss
la subida/pérdida de peso

wheat allergy
la alergia al trigo

wheelchair
la silla de ruedas

wrist
la muñeca

X-ray
la radiografía, los rayos-equis

x-ray technician
el/la técnico/a de radiografía

year
el año

yeast allergy
la alergia a la levadura

yeast infection
una infección fúngica/ (la) candidiasis

zip code
el código postal

Appendix B

Spanish-English Dictionary

a veces
sometimes

el abdomen
abdomen

el aborto
abortion

el aborto natural
miscarriage

la abrazadera hinchable
inflatable cuff

abril
April

el/la abuelo/a
grandfather/grandmother

el aceite
oil

el aerosol
nasal spray

agosto
August

el alcohol
alcohol

la alergia a la levadura
yeast allergy

la alergia a la soja
soy allergy

la alergia a las picaduras de insectos
insect sting allergy

la alergia a los animales
animal allergy

la alergia a los antibióticos
antibiotics allergy

la alergia a los cacahuetes
peanut allergy

la alergia al marisco
shellfish allergy

la alergia al polen
pollen allergy

la alergia al polvo
dust allergy

la alergia al trigo
wheat allergy

aliviar
relieve

la altura
height

las alucinaciones
hallucinations

amamantar
breastfeed

el/la amigo/a
friend

la ampolla
blister

el analgésico
analgesic

la anemia
anemia

la anestesia
anesthesia

la anestesia epidural
epidural

la anestesia local
local anesthesia

la anestesia regional or parcial
regional anesthesia

la anestesiología
anesthesiology

el/la anestesiólogo/a
anesthesiologist

el angiograma
angiogram

el anillo vaginal
ring

el año
year

la anorexia
anorexia

la ansiedad
anxiety

el antebrazo
forearm

el antiácido
antacid

el antibiótico
antibiotic

el anticoagulante
anticoagulant

el anticonvulsivante
anticonvulsant

el antidepresivo
antidepressant

el antidiarréico
antidiarrheal

el antiemético
anti-emetics

el antifúngico
antifungal

el antihipertensivo
antihypertensive

el antiinflamatorio
anti-inflammatory

el antineoplásico
antineoplastic

el antipirético
antipyretic

el antipsicótico
antipsychotic

el aparato para el suministro de oxígeno
oxygen supply device

aplicar
to apply

el ardor
burning sensation

el área de recepción
reception area

argentino/a
Argentinean

la arteriografía
arteriography

el artritis
arthritis

el ascensor (Sp.)
elevator

el/la asistente de enfermero
nurse's aid

el/la asistente de médico
physician's assistant

el asma
asthma

la aspirina
aspirin

el ataque
seizure

los ataques de pánico
panic attacks

el autismo
autism

la axila
armpit

bacterial
bacterial

el bajalengua
tongue depressor

bajo
low

el balde para pañales
pail (for diapers)

el baño
bathroom

la barbilla (Sp.)
chin

el barbitúrico
barbiturate

la bata
robe

el baumanómetro
sphygmomanometer

el biberón
bottle

la boca
mouth

boliviano/a
Bolivian

la bolsa de hielo
ice pack

el botiquín de emergencia
emergency kit

el brazo
arm

la broncoscopia
bronchoscopy

los bronquios
bronchi

la bronquitis
bronchitis

la bulimia
bulimia

el bulto
lump

buscar
look for

la cabeza
head

la cadera
hip

la cafetería
cafeteria

el cajero
cashier

la cama
bed

el cambio en el estilo de vida
change in lifestyle

los cambios en el apetito
changes in appetite

los cambios de humor/ genio
mood swings

los cambios de personalidad
personality changes

la camilla
stretcher

el cáncer
cancer

el cáncer cervical/cérvico
cervical cancer

el cáncer de ovario/ovárico
ovarian cancer

el cáncer de pecho/seno
breast cancer

la candidiasis
yeast infection

la capilla
chapel

la cápsula de gel
gel capsule

el capuchón cervical
cervical cap

la cara
face

los carbohidratos
carbohydrates

el cardiógrafo
cardiograph

la cardiología
cardiology

el/la cardiólogo/a
cardiologist

el catéter
catheter

la cateterización cardíaca
cardiac catheterization

chileno/a
Chilean

la cinta adhesiva
adhesive tape/plaster

la cintura
waist

la cirugía
surgery

la cirugía cosmética
cosmetic surgery

la cirugía curativa
curative surgery

la cirugía diagnóstica
diagnostic surgery

la cirugía de emergencia
emergency surgery

la cirugía mayor
major surgery

la cirugía menor
minor surgery

la cirugía opcional
elective surgery

la cirugía paliativa
palliative surgery

la cirugía plástica
plastic surgery

la cirugía preventiva
preventive surgery

la cirugía requerida
required surgery

la cirugía robótica
robotic surgery

el/la cirujano/a
surgeon

cistitis
urinary track infection

la cita
appointment

la ciudad
city

la clamidia
chlamydia

la codeína
codeine

el código postal
zip code

el codo
elbow

la colecistectomía
cholecystectomy

el/la colega
coworker

el colesterol alto/bajo
high/low cholesterol

colombiano/a
Colombian

el comadrón/la comadrona
midwife

el comer compulsivamente
compulsive eating

la compañía de seguros
insurance company

la complicación
complication

el comportamiento
behavior

el comportamiento catatónico
catatonic behavior

el comportamiento violento
violent behavior

el condón
male condom

el condón femenino
female condom

el/la consejero/a
counselor

el/la consejero/a pastoral
pastoral counselor

el consentimiento
consent

constante
constant

el contacto de emergencia
emergency contact

la contracción
contraction

el container
container

el correo electrónico
e-mail

costarricense
Costa Rican

la crema
gel

cuarto
fourth

cubano/a
Cuban

cubrir
cover

el cuello
neck

los cuidados intensivos
intensive care

la cuna
crib

el/la cuñado/a
brother/sister-in-law

la cureta
curette

dar a luz
to deliver

dar de alta
discharge

dar el pecho
breastfeed

dar el seno
breastfeed

de hongos
fungal

de vez en cuando
occasionally

décimo
tenth

la decisión
decision

el dedo
finger

el dedo del pie
toe

la deficiencia de memoria
memory impairment

los delirios
delusions

la demencia
dementia

la depresión
depression

depresivo
depressive

la dermatología
dermatology

el/la dermatólogo/a
dermatologist

el derrame cerebral
stroke

el descongestionante
decongestant

desmayarse
faint

el día
day

el/la diabetes
diabetes

el diafragma
diaphragm

diciembre
December

el diente
tooth

la difteria
diphtheria

la dirección
address

la displasia cervical
cervical dysplasia

disponible
available

el DIU (el dispositivo intrauterino)
IUD

doler
hurt

dolor de espalda
backache

dolor de muelas
toothache

dolor de oído
earache

los dolores del parto
labor pains

doloroso/a
painful

domingo
Sunday

dominicano/a
Dominican

el/la donante de órganos
organ donor

donar
donate

la dósis
dose

la droga para dormir
sleeping drug

las drogas
drugs

las drogas contra la ansiedad
anti-anxiety drugs

la DTaP
DTaP (diphtheria, tetanus, acellular pertussis)

la ecografía
ultrasound

ecuatoriano/a
Ecuadorian

la edad
age

el electrocardiógrafo
electrocardiograph

el electrocardiograma
EKG or ECG

el electroencefalograma
EEG

el elevador (Lat. Am.)
elevator

el email
e-mail

el embarazo
pregnancy

la endicronología
endocrinology

el/la endicronólogo/a
endocrinologist

la endoscopia
endoscopy

el enema
enema

enero
January

la enfermedad bipolar
bipolar disorder

la enfermedad de Alzheimer
Alzheimer's disease

la enfermedad de Parkinson
Parkinson's disease

la enfermedad inflamatoria pélvica
pelvic inflammatory disease

la enfermedad de tiroides
thyroid disease

las enfermedades del corazón
heart disease

el/la enfermero/a
nurse, nurse practitioner

el entumecemiento
numbness

la epilepsia
epilepsy

la episotomía
episiotomy

la escala
scale

los escalofríos
chills

la escarlatina
scarlet fever

el escudo antirradiación
radiation shield

escupir
spit

el espadadrapo
adhesive tape/plaster

la espalda
back

español/a
Spanish

el español
Spanish

el/la especialista
specialist

esperar
wait

los espermicidas vaginales
vaginal spermicides

la espinilla
shin

el espirómetro
spirometer

el/la esposo/a
husband/wife

la espuma
foam

el esputo
sputum

la esquizofrenia
schizophrenia

el estacionamiento
parking lot

el estado
state

el estado civil
marital status

estadounidense
from the United States/
American

estar
be

la esterilización femenina
female sterilization

el estetoscopio
stethoscope

el estómago
stomach

el estrés
stress

el/la estudiante de medicina
medical student

eufórico
euphoric

evacuar
have a bowel movement

el exámen pélvico
pelvic exam

examinar
examine

el excremento
stool

extirpar
remove

fallecer
die, pass

la falta de empatía
lack of empathy

la familia
family

el/la familiar
relative

el/la farmacéutico/a
pharmacist

febrero
February

la fecha
date

la fecha de nacimiento
date of birth

el fibroma uterino
uterine fibroids

la ficha del paciente
patient's chart

filipino/a
Filipino/a

la flema
phlegm

la flexibilidad
flexibility

el folleto
brochure

el formulario médico
medical form

la fortaleza muscular
muscular strength

el frasco/frasquito
container

la frente
forehead

la fuente
water fountain

fumar
smoke

la garganta
throat

la gasa esterilizada
sterilized gauze

la gastrointeritis
gastroenteritis

el gel
gel

la ginecología
gynecology

el/la ginecólogo/a
gynecologist

el glaucoma
glaucoma

la gonorrea
gonorrhea

gordo/a
fat

la gota
gout

las gotas
drops

el goteo
dripping

la grapa
staple

las grasas
fat

la gripe
influenza, flu

el grupo sanguíneo
blood type

guatemalteco/a
Guatemalan

hablar
speak

la hepatitis A, B, C
hepatitis A, B, C

el/la hermanastro/a
stepbrother/stepsister

el/la hermano/a
brother/sister

la hernia
hernia

el herpes
herpes

HiB (la meningitis)
Hib (meningitis)

el/la hijastro/a
stepson/stepsister

el/la hijo/a
son/daughter

hinchado/a
swollen

la hipertensión
hypertension

la hipnoterapia
hypnotherapy

la hipodérmica
hypodermic needle

la hipoglucemia
hypoglycemia

la histerectomía
hysterectomy

el HIV
HIV

hola
hi

hondureño/a
Honduran

la hora
hour

la hormona
hormone

el ibuprofeno
ibuprofen

la imagen por resonancia magnética
MRI

la incoherencia
incoherence

la indigestión
indigestión

la infección
infection

una infección fúngica
yeast infection

una infección genital por VPH
HPV

el inglés
English

el inhalador
inhaler

el inmunosupresor
immunosuppressant

el/la intérprete
interpreter

la intoxicación alimentaria
food poisoning

la inyección
injection

la inyección depoprovera
depo-provera injection

la IPB (el polio)
IPB (polio)

la irritabilidad
irritability

irritable
irritable

la irritación
irritation

la jalea de petróleo
petroleum jelly

el jarabe
syrup

la jeringa, la jeringuilla
syringe

jueves
Thursday

el juicio afectado
impaired judgment

julio
July

junio
June

el labio
lip

el laboratorio
laboratory

la laparoscopia
laparoscopic surgery

la laringitis
laryngitis

lavar
wash

el laxativo, el laxante
laxative

la lengua
tongue

el lenguaje desorganizado
disorganized speech

la leucemia
leukemia

la libra
pound

la ligadura tubárica
tubal litigation

el limpiador
cleanser

limpiar, limpio/a
clean

las llagas
sores

llamar
call

la loción
lotion

el lugar de empleo
place of employment

lunes
Monday

el lupus
lupus

la madrastra
stepfather/stepmother

la madre
mother

el mamograma
mammogram

la mandíbula
jaw

la mano
hand

mareado/a
dizzy

martes
Tuesday

el martillo de reflejos
reflex hammer

marzo
March

la mastectomía
mastectomy

masticar
to chew

mayo
May

la medicación
medication

la medicina
medicine

la medicina antiarrítmica
antiarrhythmic

la medicina antiviral
antiviral

medir
measure

la mejilla
cheek

mejorar
improve

la meningitis
meningitis

la menopausia
menopause

menor de edad
minor

la menstruación
menstruation

el mentón (Lat. Am.)
chin

el mes
month

meter
insert

el método del ritmo
fertility awareness/
rhythm method

mexicano/a
Mexican

la microcirugía
microsurgery

el microcronómetro
timer

el microscopio
microscope

miércoles
Wednesday

la migraña
migraine

los minerales
minerals

el minuto
minute

moderadamente
moderately

el moisés
bassinet

el monitor
monitor

el monitor del electro-cardiograma
ECG monitor

la morfina
morphine

la mucosidad
mucus

la muestra
sample

las muletas
crutches

la muñeca
wrist

el muslo
thigh

la nalga
buttocks

la nariz
nose

necesitar
need

negativo/a
negative

la neumonía
pneumonia

la neurología
neurology

el/la neurólogo/a
neurologist

nicarangüense
Nicaraguan

el/la nieto/a
grandson/granddaughter

el no poder dormir
inability to sleep

el nombre
name

normal
normal

noveno
ninth

noviembre
November

el/la novio/a
boyfriend/girlfriend

la nuera
daughter-in-law

el número
number

el número de la seguro social
social security number

el número de teléfono
phone number

nunca
never

la nutrición
nutrition

el/la nutricionista
nutritionist

obeso/a
fat

observar
observe

el/la obstetra
obstetrician

la obstetricia
obstetrics

octavo
eighth

octubre
October

la oftalmología
ophthalmology

el/la oftalmólogo/a
ophthalmologist

el oftalmoscopio
ophthalmoscope

el oído
ear (internal)

el ojo
eye

oler, el olor
smell

la oncología
oncology

el/la oncólogo/a
oncologist

la onza
ounce

la operación
surgery

la operación cesárea
cesarean section

la operación de láser
laser surgery

operar
operate

la oreja
ear (external)

*los órganos reproducti-
vos*
reproductive organs

el orinal
bedpan

orinar
urinate

la ortopedia
orthopedics

el/la ortopedista
orthopaedist

la osteoporosis
osteoporosis

*el/la otorrino-laringólo-
go/a*
otorhinolaryngologist

el ovario
ovary

el/la paciente
patient

el padrastro
stepfather/stepmother

el padre
father

los palitos de algodón
cotton swabs

el pañal
diaper

panameño/a
Panamanian

el parche
patch

el parche anticonceptivo
birth control patch

el/la pariente/a
relative

parir
to deliver

el Parkinsons
Parkinson's disease

la paroditis, las paperas
mumps

el parto
delivery

la pastilla
tablet, pill

payaguayo/a
Paraguayan

la PCV
PCV (pneumococcal
conjugate vaccine)

el pecho
chest, breast

el/la pediatra
pediatrician

pegar
to attach

el pene
penis

*los pensamientos de
muerte repetidos*
recurring thoughts of
death

la pérdida de energía
loss of energy

*la pérdida de estribos
frecuente*
frequent loss of temper

la pérdida de memoria
memory loss

*las perforaciones en los
órganos*
punctured organs

el periodo
menstruation

el permiso
permission

peruano/a
Peruvian

pesar
weigh

el peso
weight, scale

el pezón
nipple

picar
itch

el picor
itchiness

el pie
foot

las piedras en el riñón
kidney stones

la piel
skin

la pierna
leg

la píldora
pill

*la píldora del día
después*
ECP emergency contra-
ceptive pills

la pipera
pipette

el piso
floor

la placenta
placenta

la planta del pie
sole

el polio
polio

poner
to put

el porcentaje de grasa del cuerpo
body fat percentage

positivo
positive

el preservativo masculino
male condom

la presión sanguínea alta/baja
high/low blood pressure

presionar
pressure

primer
first

el/la primo/a
male cousin/female cousin

la profesión
occupation

el/la prometido/a
fiancé/fiancée

proteger
protect

las proteínas
protein

el/la psicoanalista
psychoanalyst

el/la psicólogo/a
psychologist

la psicoterapia
psychotherapy

el/la psiquiatra
psychiatrist

la psiquiatría
psychiatry

puertorriqueño/a
Puerto Rican

el pulgar
thumb

los puntos, las puntadas
stitches

el pulso en descanso
resting heart rate

la quimoterapia
chemotherapy

quinto
fifth

unos quistes en el ovario
ovarian cysts

la radiografía
X-ray

la radiología
radiology

el/la radiólogo/a
radiologist

rara vez
rarely

los rayos-equis
X-ray

la reacción
reaction

las reacciones alérgicas
allergic reactions

la recepción
reception area

el/la recepcionista
receptionist

los recursos
resources

el relajante de músculos
muscle relaxant

el remedio contra el resfriado
cold remedy

los remedios naturales
natural remedies

reposicionar
restore

la resistencia física
endurance

respirar
breath

el resultado
result

el riesgo
risk

rociar
to spray

la rodilla
knee

romper la bolsa de agua
break water

la rubeóla
German measles

sábado
Saturday

la sala de emergencia
emergency room

la sala de espera
waiting room

la sala de maternidad
maternity ward

la sala principal
main lobby

la sala de recuperación
recovery room

la salida
exit

la salida de emergencia
emergency exit

la saliva
saliva

salvadoreño/a
El Salvadoran

el salpullido
rash

sangrar
to bleed

el sangrar excesivamente
excessive bleeding

sano/a, saludable
healthy

el sarampión
measles

las secreciones vaginales
vaginal discharge

el/la secretario/a
secretary

la sedación consciente or intravenosa
conscious or intravenous sedation

la sedación excesiva
over-sedation

el sedativo
sedative

segundo
second

el seguro médico
insurance

la semana
week

el seno
breast

la sensación de calor intenso
hot flashes

los sentimientos de impotencia
feelings of helplessness

septiembre
September

séptimo
seventh

ser
be

los servicios (Sp.)
bathrooms

sexto
sixth

el SIDA
AIDS

la sífilis
syphilis

los signos vitales
vital signs

la silla alta
high chair

la silla de ruedas
wheelchair

la sinusitis
sinusitis

el sistema circulatorio
circulatory system

el sistema digestivo
digestive system

el sistema endocrino
endocrine system

el sistema gastrointestinal
gastrointestinal system

el sistema nervioso
nervous system

el sistema reproductivo
reproductive system

el sistema respiratorio
respiratory system

el sobaco
armpit

el/la sobrino/a
nephew/niece

la sonda
catheter

el spray
nasal spray

la subida/pérdida de peso
weight gain/loss

sudar
sweat

los sudores nocturnos
night sweats

el/la suegro/a
father-in-law/mother-in-law

el supositorio
suppository

el supresor de tos
cough suppressant

la tableta efervescente
effeverescent table

la tableta masticable
chewtab

el talco
powder

el talón
heel

la taquicardia
tachycardia

TDAH (el transtorno por déficit de atención con hiperactividad)
ADHD

el/la técnico/a de radiografía
x-ray technician

el teléfono
telephone

tener
have

tener arcadas
gag

la tensión sanguínea
blood pressure

el/la terapeuta
therapist

el/la terapeuta físico
physical therapist

el/la terapeuta de lenguaje
speech therapist

la terapia de comportamiento
behavior therapy

la terapia electroconvulsiva
electroconvulsive therapy

la terapia física
physical therapy

la terapia con medicamentos
drug therapy

la terapia de radiación
radiation theraphy

tercer
third

el termómetro
thermometer

el testículo
testicle

el tétanos
tetanus

la tetina, el chupón
nipple (on a bottle)

la tía
aunt

el tío
uncle

el timbre
call bell

la tiña
ringworm

el/la titular de la póliza
policy holder

el tobillo
ankle

tocar
touch

todo el tiempo
all the time

todos los días
daily

tomar
to take

la tomografía computerizada
computed tomography or CT scan

el torniquete
tourniquet

la tos ferina
pertussis

toser
cough

el/la trabajador/a social
social worker

tragar
swallow

el tranquilizante
tranquilizer

la transfusión de sangre
blood transfusion

transplantar, el transplante
transplant

el transtorno de ansiedad generalizada
anxiety disorder

el transtorno de comportamiento obsesivo compulsivo
obsessive compulsive behavior disorder

el transtorno de estrés postraumático
PTSD, post-traumatic stress disorder

el transtorno de personalidad
personality disorder

el tratamiento
treatment

los tratamientos alternativos
alternative treatments

el tratamiento experimental
experimental treatment

la tristeza
sadness

las trompas de falopio
fallopian tubes

la tuberculosis
tuberculosis, TB

la úlcera
ulcer

el ultrasound
ultrasound

la uña
nail

el ungüento
ointment

la urología
urology

el/la urólogo/a
urologist

la urticaria
hives

uruguayo/a
Uruguayan

el útero
uterus

la vagina
vagina

la varicela
varicella (chicken pox)

la vasectomía
vasectomy

el/la vecino/a
neighbor

la venda
bandage

venezolano
Venezuelan

ver
see

las verrugas
warts

viernes
Friday

vírica
viral

la vitamina
vitamin

el yerno
son-in law

INDEX